Gregory B. Collins, MD
Thomas L. Culbertson, DMin, PhD

Mental Illness
and Psychiatric Treatment
A Guide for Pastoral Counselors

Pre-publication
REVIEWS,
COMMENTARIES,
EVALUATIONS . . .

"**G**iven the enormous amount of contact that clergy have with emotionally troubled people of all ages, it is surprising how little has been written to help them understand the complexity of modern day care of the mentally troubled. This book does a very thorough job of rectifying this deficiency. Adopting a holistic approach to pastoral care, it gives pastors a 'grand tour' of the field of psychiatry and its related disciplines of clinical psychology and counseling. Written with clarity and without excessive technical jargon, it not only provides clergy with a broad overview of the major disorders, but also gives special emphasis to the knowledge and skills pastors must develop to be effective in identifying, supporting, and referring those in special need to the appropriate mental health professional.

One particular feature of the book that gives it special value is the substantial inclusion of relevant case examples that help to put a face and feeling to the hard facts and descriptive symptomology of mental illness. Each story is almost like doing 'grand rounds' with a master clinician who points out where and how a pastor can counsel, support, and point sufferers toward spiritual resources to aid their healing. The book maintains a strong emphasis throughout on the spiritual needs of those struggling with emotional problems. It can be used as required reading for those in training for the ministry, not just those specializing in pastoral counseling."

Archibald D. Hart, PhD, FPPR
Senior Professor of Psychology
and Dean Emeritus,
Graduate School of Psychology,
Fuller Theological Seminary,
Pasadena, CA; Executive Editor,
American Association
of Christian Counselors

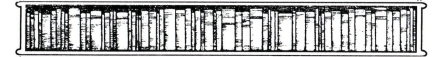

The Haworth Pastoral Press®
An Imprint of The Haworth Press, Inc.
New York • London • Oxford

Mental Illness and Psychiatric Treatment
A Guide for Pastoral Counselors

THE HAWORTH PASTORAL PRESS
Religion and Mental Health
Harold G. Koenig, MD
Senior Editor

Understanding Clergy Misconduct in Religious Systems: Scapegoating, Family Secrets, and the Abuse of Power by Candace R. Benyei

What the Dying Teach Us: Lessons on Living by Samuel Lee Oliver

The Pastor's Family: The Challenges of Family Life and Pastoral Responsibilities by Daniel L. Langford

Somebody's Knocking at Your Door: AIDS and the African-American Church by Ronald Jeffrey Weatherford and Carole Boston Weatherford

Grief Education for Caregivers of the Elderly by Junietta Baker McCall

The Obsessive-Compulsive Disorder: Pastoral Care for the Road to Change by Robert M. Collie

The Pastoral Care of Children by David H. Grossoehme

Ways of the Desert: Becoming Holy Through Difficult Times by William F. Kraft

Caring for a Loved One with Alzheimer's Disease: A Christian Perspective by Elizabeth T. Hall

"Martha, Martha": How Christians Worry by Elaine Leong Eng

Spiritual Care for Children Living in Specialized Settings: Breathing Underwater by Michael F. Friesen

Broken Bodies, Healing Hearts: Reflections of a Hospital Chaplain by Gretchen W. TenBrook

Shared Grace: Therapists and Clergy Working Together by Marion Bilich, Susan Bonfiglio, and Steven Carlson

The Pastor's Guide to Psychiatric Disorders and Mental Health Resources by W. Brad Johnson and William L. Johnson

Pastoral Counseling: A Gestalt Approach by Ward A. Knights

Christ-Centered Therapy: Empowering the Self by Russ Harris

Bioethics from a Faith Perspective: Ethics in Health Care for the Twenty-First Century by Jack Hanford

Family Abuse and the Bible: The Scriptural Perspective by Aimee K. Cassidy-Shaw

When the Caregiver Becomes the Patient: A Journey from a Mental Disorder to Recovery and Compassionate Insight by Daniel L. Langford and Emil J. Authelet

A Theology of God-Talk: The Language of the Heart by J. Timothy Allen

A Practical Guide to Hospital Ministry: Healing Ways by Junietta B. McCall

Pastoral Care for Post-Traumatic Stress Disorder: Healing the Shattered Soul by Daléne Fuller Rogers

Integrating Spirit and Psyche: Using Women's Narratives in Psychotherapy by Mary Pat Henehan

Chronic Pain: Biomedical and Spiritual Approaches by Harold G. Koenig

Spirituality in Pastoral Counseling and the Community Helping Professions by Charles Topper

Parish Nursing: A Handbook for the New Millennium edited by Sybil D. Smith

Mental Illness and Psychiatric Treatment: A Guide for Pastoral Counselors by Gregory B. Collins and Thomas Culbertson

Mental Illness and Psychiatric Treatment
A Guide for Pastoral Counselors

Gregory B. Collins, MD
Thomas Culbertson, DMin, PhD

The Haworth Pastoral Press®
An Imprint of The Haworth Press, Inc.
New York • London • Oxford

Published by

The Haworth Pastoral Press®, an imprint of The Haworth Press, Inc., 10 Alice Street, Binghamton, NY 13904-1580.

PUBLISHER'S NOTE
Identities and circumstances of individuals discussed in this book have been changed to protect confidentiality.

Cover design by Bridget Parlato.

Library of Congress Cataloging-in-Publication Data

Collins, Gregory B.
    Mental illness and psychiatric treatment : a guide for pastoral counselors / Gregory B. Collins, Thomas Culbertson.
        p. cm.
    Includes bibliographical references and index.
    ISBN 0-7890-1879-9 (hardcover : alk. paper)—ISBN 0-7890-1880-2 (softcover : alk. paper)
    1. Mentally ill—Pastoral counseling of. I. Culbertson, Thomas. II. Title.

BV4461 .C65 2003
259' .42—dc21
                                                                          2002015167

To Reverend Ronald Morgan, Director Emeritus,
Clinical Pastoral Education Program,
The Cleveland Clinic Foundation,
who showed us daily how pastoral services can
enrich and assist in the healing process
for the emotionally troubled

To our patients and congregants, who through
their daily lives of triumph and suffering
have taught us so much

To hospital chaplains everywhere,
whose calling is unique

ABOUT THE AUTHORS

Gregory B. Collins, MD, is Medical Director and Section Head of the Alcohol and Drug Recovery Center in the Department of Psychiatry and Psychology at The Cleveland Clinic Foundation. Dr. Collins was formerly on the faculty of the Ashland Theological Seminary, where he lectured on psychiatric topics for clergy. He has held faculty positions at Ohio State University, Georgetown University, and Case Western Reserve University. In his clinical practice, Dr. Collins has seen well over 30,000 patients. He has an eclectic and holistic treatment philosophy that is aimed at the restoration of body, mind, spirit, and social supports. He incorporates a wide variety of spiritual resources in his methodology, borrowing heavily from Christian, Judaic, Islamic, and Eastern religious traditions, in addition to scientific, medical, and socio-psychological interventions. Dr. Collins is the recipient of The Cleveland Clinic Foundation Bernard Loeschen Pastoral Care Award for "excellence as an advocate, consultant, and teacher, and for exemplifying spiritual care in his person and profession." Dr. Collins lives with his wife in Solon, Ohio, and has three children.

The Rev. Thomas L. Culbertson, DMin, PhD, is Rector of the Emmanuel Episcopal Church, a large urban congregation in Baltimore, Maryland. Dr. Culbertson's academic-pastoral work includes clinical pastoral education, ministerial courses in psychiatry, and clinical work in alcohol rehabilitation. Along with these endeavors, his parish ministry includes serving as Chair of the diocesan-wide advisory committee for a drug and alcohol rehabilitation program on-site at his parish, membership on the committee for oversight of the Episcopal Chaplaincy at Johns Hopkins Hospital, and membership on the board of Baltimore's Clinical Pastoral Education Program. Commensurate with these interests is a vital concern with the methods and rationale used by parish clergy in their counseling. Dr. Culbertson is married, with two grown daughters and a grandson.

CONTENTS

Foreword

The position and role of the pastor, whether a minister, priest, rabbi, or imam, is clearly unique in American society. No other person carries quite the same combination of authority and caring. Consequently, no other person carries the same responsibility for (and is expected to have the ability to respond to) the troubled and the suffering. This is especially true in the pastor's role with the mentally ill. At the same time, no other group of persons under the pastor's care has left him or her feeling so unhelpful and inadequate.

As every pastor knows, no congregation is exempt from mental illness, regardless of size, location, denomination, or theological or liturgical orientation. At the same time, the stigma surrounding mentally ill persons, although it has eased some in recent years, still remains strong across all elements of society. Too often the early signs of mental illness are denied or rationalized, or they are simply not understood as symptoms at all. Often the situation deteriorates over months or years and then presents in the pastor's office when the breaking point occurs. No wonder pastors feel so overwhelmed and inadequate in this crisis. In a real sense, they are. Pastors who have picked up this book for this reason should take heart. It is a significant resource in responding to this calling.

Gregory Collins, a practicing psychiatrist, and Thomas Culbertson, the pastor of an active urban congregation, have provided pastors with a working knowledge of psychiatry and the major psychiatric disorders. In clear, nontechnical language and a down-to-earth attitude, they provide pastors with the information they need and a counseling process that can be followed in ministering to those with mental and emotional disorders. In addition, they give concrete advice about what role to fill or what words to say in particular circumstances and warn about some of the pitfalls that are unique to clergy. Finally, the authors provide an up-to-date bibliography for further reading.

On the other hand, this is not a textbook in psychiatry or the specialized field of professional pastoral counseling. Nor is it a how-to book that will make the pastor a professional therapist for the mentally ill. The authors provide a means of understanding those emotionally disturbed persons who often reach out to the leader of a spiritual community and explain how to proceed in this difficult area of pastoral care and counseling, an area that is often overlooked or too briefly treated in theological education.

Each chapter provides case illustrations of the lives of people burdened with a particular mental illness. Pastors may recognize many correspondences among their congregants. The book's style gives a feeling of being in consultation with Dr. Collins and Dr. Culbertson, discussing a case that has been brought to them for advice. Pastors will return again and again to these pages as a resource in particular relationships and as a guide for further reading and study. As in all conversations, not all topics are covered, and those that are may have differing levels of attention; nor will this conversation answer all questions that pastors may have, although it may raise some that had not been previously considered. But it will certainly encourage and empower pastors to engage in their role as a counseling pastor to the mentally ill with more confidence and effectiveness.

In addition to their words, the authors, like good counselors, provide a nonverbal element as well: demonstration of a collaboration between a psychiatrist and a pastor. It models an appreciation between the disciplines of psychiatry and religion that have for so long been at war with each other. This model may encourage pastors to establish such a collaborative relationship, to seek out a psychiatrist, psychologist, or other mental health professional in their community to serve as a resource in ministering to the mentally ill. This book will serve as a good introduction to disorders to discuss, and pastors will find their ministries enhanced and enriched.

The Reverend Barrett Rudd
Retired Chaplain
Sheppard Pratt Hospital
Baltimore, Maryland

Preface and Acknowledgments

The idea for this book arose from lectures at the Cleveland Psychiatric Institute to students in an advanced pastoral counseling course of the Ashland Theological Seminary. It is the product of a long and mutually rewarding collaboration between Gregory B. Collins, MD, a psychiatrist who was then a faculty member of the seminary, and the Reverend Thomas L. Culbertson, DMin, PhD, who was, at that time, a doctoral student and active clergyman.

Based on their experiences in this pastoral counseling curriculum, the authors became aware of the growing interest on the part of religious professionals in working with emotionally troubled and mentally ill people. This book is designed to bring knowledge and skills to the religious professional who seeks to provide special ministry to the emotionally troubled. While this is not an attempt to turn clergy into psychiatrists, the authors do believe that a basic understanding of psychiatric illnesses, theory, and treatment modalities can only enlarge the perspective of the pastoral worker. The pastor can thereby occupy a rightful and important place on the holistic health care team, with the goal of restoring vitality of body, mind, and spirit to the person suffering from emotional illness.

We gratefully acknowledge the help and encouragement of so many who contributed in countless ways to this manuscript: the staff of The Cleveland Clinic Foundation, our typists Joan Kocka and Audrey Renz; the people of St. Paul's Episcopal Church of Cleveland Heights, Ohio; the people of Emmanuel Episcopal Church in Baltimore, Maryland; the spiritual and editorial mentoring of Reverend Ronald Morgan; and our loving and ever-patient spouses, Denise Collins and Deborah Culbertson.

Introduction

The Function of Pastoral Care in a Holistic Health Approach

In our collective experience with thousands of patients and parishioners with a variety of psychiatric disorders, we have repeatedly observed that the person is sick in toto, i.e., in mind, body, and spirit. In addition, his or her social milieu often is profoundly disturbed, with legal problems, divorce, insolvency, and even homelessness. Because of the global nature of these emotional disturbances, this book addresses the clergy's role in a holistic team approach to the treatment of emotional illnesses. We believe that appropriate, knowledgeable pastoral counseling has a significant place in the treatment of the emotionally troubled person. We believe that emotional illnesses, as with other illnesses, are complex disorders that primarily require professional, expert management. Yet the pastoral counselor, in cooperation with the psychiatrist, can do much to assist in the recovery process. At the very least, the pastoral counselor, as part of a multidisciplinary team, can bring to the emotionally troubled person sensitivity, understanding, and measured patience. At a more advanced level, the minister can recognize and define as spiritual symptoms of disease any negative, inappropriate, or self-defeating attitudes or behaviors. The minister, priest, rabbi, or imam can thus deal more specifically with these manifestations of illness through pastoral intervention and counseling.

In our estimation, spiritual illness is a dimension of emotional illness. We have frequently observed that severe emotional or psychiatric illnesses often involve spiritual sickness as well. Spiritual sickness is a complex concept that may take many forms depending on the type of emotional illness. For example, a severe depressive illness might involve loss of faith, abandonment of hope, loss of a right relationship with God, or even self-hatred, guilt, despair, and self-annihilation. A psychotic reaction marked by loss of contact with reality might involve abnormal self-importance, grandiosity, fear, or stubbornly mistaken perceptions of reality. A problem with alcoholism might involve violent behavior, irresponsible conduct, denial of loss of control over liquor, or abject guilt, shame, and self-hatred. The personality disorders may involve profound disturbances in social relationships and conduct characterized by self-centered anger, impulsiveness, dishonesty, manipulation, or distrust of others. The anxious states might involve loss of faith or trust in God, obsessive fears and tensions, or inability to turn things over to God's divine care. These are common components of emotional disturbance that are amenable to pastoral intervention as part of the patient's treatment program.

We expand on these themes in this book, focusing on specific types of emotional illness with pastoral intervention in mind. Our goal is to be as helpful as possible to the practicing member of the clergy who is called upon to offer pastoral support or to intervention for an emotionally troubled person. We will attempt to focus on specific, observable phenomena. Theoretical concepts and approaches will be of secondary concern, and these are presented only briefly to afford the clergy some historical background and additional understanding of the psychiatric components of these illnesses and their treatments.

Our format is designed to help the pastor grasp the principles of intervention in each of these categories of disorders. Each clinical chapter therefore follows a four-part format: (1) recognition of the disorder, (2) assessment of severity, (3) crisis intervention, and (4) counseling in the recovery phase. These four areas cover the duties and responsibilities of the clergyperson as part of the holistic health care team.

Only recently has there been renewed appreciation of the holistic nature of emotional and physical illnesses, and of the necessity for appropriate multidisciplinary treatment. In earlier times, psychiatric illnesses were thought to result from witchcraft, possession by demons, or sinfulness, but with the evolution of scientific medicine these notions were abandoned. In their haste to be scientific, however, modern practitioners of medicine and psychiatry may have overlooked the important role of spiritual health and the value of pastoral intervention in sustaining and restoring emotional stability.

Modern psychiatry has its roots in the practice of physical medicine, that is, in neurology, the study of the nervous system. Modern psychiatry essentially was born with the discovery that some patients who were paralyzed yet showed no demonstrable neurologic disease could be helped to walk and function normally with a few brief sessions of hypnosis and hypnotic suggestion. Although this susceptibility to hypnotic suggestion was originally thought to be due to neurologic peculiarities, Freud and other early investigators soon discovered that these patients' symptoms resulted from hidden psychological ailments, which, when exposed through hypnotherapy or psychoanalysis, could be discovered and removed. Thus, from an early interest in neurologic illness, modern psychiatry began to focus more intently on the illness of the "mind," with problems and treatments of a psychological nature. Only recently has modern psychiatry come full circle to the realization that the spiritual aspect is just as important a component of the total person as are the mind and body.

The religious world never lost sight of the spiritual elements in human nature, for the religious community has always served as a repository of spiritual health and recovery for humankind. Through the practice and application of religious principles, rituals, scripture, and community life, religion offered the structure for recovery from spiritual problems. Yet just as modern scientific psychiatry has often omitted the spiritual aspects in its quest to heal the whole person, so too were severely troubled individuals not always adequately assisted solely by pastoral interventions. We all owe a great debt of gratitude to the self-help movement, and in particular to Alcoholics Anonymous, for the discovery that alcoholism involves illness of mind, body, and spirit, and also for developing a therapeutic framework integrating physical, psychological, and spiritual recovery. Experience has shown that other types of emotional disturbances involve physical, psychological, and spiritual problems as well, and that truly comprehensive assistance to the emotionally troubled person involves attention to all of these areas.

This holistic approach to the emotionally troubled person is not an entirely new concept. The best psychotherapy has always embodied the expression or endorsement of some spiritual or moral values, although many psychiatrists themselves might be uncomfortable with the assertion that they are, in fact, practicing moral or value-based psychotherapy. In practice, that is actually what often happens. Indeed, psychiatrists are legally charged by society with the prevention or treatment of violent or self-destructive tendencies in the mentally ill. Certainly the prevention of such acts is a moral good. The goal of treatment is for the emotionally disturbed person to learn to function at a higher level or to adhere to a standard of right and wrong in his or her thinking, attitudes, emotions, and behaviors. In the same way, a good deal of ministerial counseling is, in fact, psychotherapy without being labeled as such. Emotionally troubled people often identify their needs as spiritual or pastoral, rather than as psychiatric or psychological, and often the pastor is the first person to whom the troubled patient or family member turns for help. These situations afford the religious professional an opportunity for real participation in the holistic process of recovery of the troubled individual.

What do we mean by "the emotionally troubled person"? How can we define emotional illness or disturbance? The focus of this book is not so much the person with a brief, time-limited crisis or problem, who comes equipped with a useful array of coping skills to see him or her through and back to a "normal" baseline. Rather, our focus is on chronic, long-lasting, severely disabling conditions with not only an acute crisis component but also an enduring failure to reestablish a normal, adaptive condition. Such illnesses are often difficult to define or recognize in that they do not resemble physical illnesses such as tumors, which can be seen on X ray, or microorganisms, which appear under a microscope. Sometimes physical or chemical changes are present, but in most cases they are not discernible. Most cases of emotional disturbance, however, do involve personality changes. These changes are usually "unhealthy" in that they involve less responsibility, productivity, contentment, stability, judgment, satisfaction, community, or spiritual connection. The affected individual may complain about feeling bad, "not feeling like myself," or having diminished energy. Symptoms of depression and anxiety, or disturbances of thinking and behavior, are distressing to the person and/or those around him or her. Usual routines are disrupted, and behavior may be unpredictable, bizarre, even destructive. Often there is social withdrawal and alienation characterized by anger and pathological self-absorption. Spiritual isolation and impoverishment are frequently seen. The emotionally troubled person usually comes to a distressed or crisis state, usually as a result of failing to function normally in meeting his or her needs or in caring for routine responsibilities.

Thus, the emotionally troubled person often presents a complex matrix of problems, including pathological thoughts, inappropriate actions, impaired social interactions, and spiritual isolation. What, then, is the function of pastoral care for such a person? We believe that to be truly effective in caring for the holistic needs of congregants, the minister may have to call into play at appropriate times her or his role as either long-term counselor or sacramental officiant. Each function has value, but neither is fully adequate to deal with the broad spectrum of problems presented by the emotionally troubled. A much more successful and fulfilling ministry is likely if the sacerdotal role and pastoral counseling are part of an integrated, holistic team approach. The professional enrichment in this approach frees the pastor from isolation, frustration, and mediocrity. A holistic approach wherein the pastor works in conjunction with others on the health care team is often the means to both a more fulfilling ministry and to more competent care for the troubled person.

Resistance to a holistic team approach may surface for any number of reasons, including self-imposed professional isolation. Often there is a professional inclination to work alone and, hence, a sense of professional teamwork is often lacking. This is not entirely the pastor's fault; he or she often must overcome the isolation of pastoral life from so-called secular life. But we encourage pastors to view themselves as part of the larger social community, especially in the health care area. Such a view implies a larger role of the pastor in the recovery process. An isolationist's professional stance involves a narrow interpretation of pastoral duties, emphasizing sacerdotal tasks, perhaps to the exclusion of other restorative tools. An isolationist's stance could be limited to praying over the mentally ill or making such statements as, "God is the only answer." To be a truly effective holistic health care team member, the pastor must develop skills for addressing the problems of the whole person. He or she must be open to a more interactive relationship with a troubled person and must not be limited to a ritualistic function. The pastor is often the first person to whom people turn in moments of crisis or upheaval. He or she, therefore, should know as much as possible about the kinds of disorders that befall people and be prepared with a sensitive ear and unprejudiced understanding. He or she should have knowledge of a human condition from both a religious and a psychological prospective. The pastor should develop a skilled listening ear that is sensitive to the spiritual component of emotional health. Such listening is both an art and an acquired skill. Interest, involvement, and empathy are hallmarks of such skilled listening. A skilled listener conveys an unspoken message of caring and concern, as well as willingness to help. But listening alone is not enough.

In the process of listening, our concern must also include the familial and societal structures surrounding the person under pastoral care. His or her relationship to those structures should be explored to see where and how the counselee fits into his or her world. Having a composite picture of the person seeking pastoral help is absolutely necessary in the design of a continuing care program. A well-rounded picture of the counselee is essential if the pastor is to help in achieving meaningful goals. By understanding this social matrix, the pastor can help the person make appropriate decisions regarding his or her future, bearing in mind that the best outcome may require access to ongoing therapeutic supervision.

Initially, the healing process is characterized by eliciting information and emotion. Gradually, the person is moved from understanding to acceptance to purposeful self-improvement. Courage to act or to accept change must sometimes come through the pastor. He or she can help break through misdirected self-will to help the person gain stability and growth. The pastor may be the vehicle for this spiritual intervention so that the person under care can be directed to take responsibility for his or her own life. Movement from upheaval and chaos to order and healthy self-direction is an appropriate goal for the pastor in the counseling relationship.

We also suggest that an essential component in holistic pastoral care is the process of referral. The ability to recognize the right moment to suggest further help is important because the person under care has placed trust in the pastor. Reassurance that the pastor's support will continue is always advisable. The common goal of pastor and professional counselor in the treatment process is a healthy, nonsuffering, functional person. The tools and skills of a psychiatrist may lead religious people out of darkness into a more abundant relationship with themselves, the world, and God. The suffering person's quest for spiritual fulfillment can indeed be recognized and facilitated by the holistic psychiatrist. Professional therapists who are sensitive to this religious aspect of the whole person can be most helpful in the process of change, reintegration, and growth. Pastors should have a list of competent professional therapists to whom they can refer. The object of referral is not necessarily the matching of religious convictions of the counselee and counselor, unless concern for matching is raised by the patient. Rather, referral is based on concern for the kind of expertise needed, for example, psychiatrist, marriage counselor, child psychologist, and the like. Pastors should follow up on their referrals by asking the psychiatrist what progress has been made and how they can continue to be of assistance. A skilled psychiatrist will have very little hesitation in offering suggestions for helpful pastoral intervention. Pastors' willingness to refer means that they are already part of a larger health care process. In a collaborative, interprofessional design, the pastor and mental health professional are both aware of the contributions of religion and the health sciences in achieving emotional stability and productive living. Their mutual hope should be Isaiah's hope: "Then shall blind men's eyes be opened, and the ears of the deaf be unstopped. Then shall the lame man leap like a deer, and the tongue of the dumb shout aloud" (Isaiah 35:5-6 New English Bible).

Chapter 1

An Overview of Psychiatry

To be part of the holistic health care team, the pastor must have a working knowledge of how the other team members function. That is, she or he must be familiar with basic psychiatric terminology and have some understanding of the many therapeutic modalities employed by the practicing psychiatrist. Meeting the need for a comprehensive overview of psychiatry, however, is a difficult undertaking, one that itself would require a very large book. Psychiatric illnesses are too numerous to be cataloged here, and diagnostic symptoms are extremely variable. No two patients are exactly alike in their presentation of signs and symptoms. Also, modern psychiatry combines a good deal of art and science in ways that are difficult to describe, quantify, or validate. In no other specialities of medicine are there so many theoretical diversities and so many schools of treatment. One reasonable approach to understanding this complex subject is through history. Although the following material is far from a complete historical review, it should provide a basic understanding of some psychiatric fundamentals. These fundamentals provide the theoretical basis for the study and practice of modern psychiatry. Many of these concepts or ideas have become so popularized that educated laypeople will understand them immediately. The interested pastor should study these fundamental principles and have a ready, if basic, understanding of them. They do provide at least one framework with which to view and understand our human nature, with its vulnerability to mental illness.

HISTORY OF PSYCHIATRY

There can be little question that modern psychiatry began with the contributions of Sigmund Freud. Indeed, prior to Freud, there was scarcely a science of psychiatry at all and virtually no understanding of normal mental processes, much less of mental disorders. Freud's observations and subsequent writings drastically revolutionized our understanding of how the mind works in health and in sickness. He and his colleagues were largely responsible for the first successful "talking cures," and his writings on mental processes have popularized psychoanalytic concepts to such a remarkable extent that they are indeed almost household words.

Sigmund Freud was born to a Jewish family in 1856 in what is now the Czech Republic. At an early age, Freud moved with his family to Vienna, where he lived until 1938, when the Nazis took over Austria and he was forced to flee to England. As a student, Freud was strongly influenced by the scientific thinkers of the day, and he cultivated qualities of scientific discipline and intellectual integrity. Freud's early medical training demonstrated his marked interest in brain function and psychology, and he postulated a physical relationship between psychological phenomena and physical events in the brain cells. Early in his career, Freud began to study neurology. In 1885 he was the recipient of a traveling grant to study for nineteen weeks in Paris at the Salpetriere Hospital under the great French neurologist Charcot. Freud was impressed with Charcot's work with hysteria, an illness characterized by weakness, paralysis, or sensory losses such as blindness, deafness, or numbness, all without demonstrable neurologic pathology. Freud became convinced that hysterics were suffering from real illness and were not malingering or faking, as was the widespread belief of the day. Charcot, through the use of hypnosis, was able to precipitate hysterical paralyses, seizures, and other typical symptoms, and Freud began to believe that such illnesses were, in fact, psychological. Freud subsequently studied hypnosis in France and was deeply impressed with the results that French physicians were able to obtain. He was also fascinated by previously hidden mental processes that could be examined under hypnosis. He returned to Vienna in 1886 with the intention of practicing neurology. He did so and published several highly regarded papers on neurological subjects. By 1887, Freud had become interested in the various psychological phenomena that he was seeing as part of his practice, and he became friends with Josef Breuer, another Viennese physician.

Breuer and Freud eventually published "Studies on Hysteria," which was largely inspired by Breuer's work with "Anna O," a twenty-one-year-old girl. Anna, an intelligent girl who had been deeply devoted to her father, for two years suffered a debilitating illness with symptoms of severe paralysis and numbness in both legs, disturbance of eye movements, impairment of vision, difficulty in maintaining head position, nervous cough, nausea when eating, and intense thirst yet loss of power to swallow liquids. Her ability to speak diminished until she could neither speak nor understand German, her native language. She frequently had states of "absence" or delirium during which her entire personality altered. Anna's illness first began while she was caring for her beloved father during his eventually fatal illness. She was forced to abandon this task because of her own illness. Sympathetic observation soon enabled Breuer to note that she usually mumbled some words during her absence states. Breuer put her into a hypnotic trance and repeated these words to her, and she was eventually able to reexperience the thoughts that were characteristic of the absences. These thoughts were like reveries or daydreams, which usually began with a girl beside her father's sickbed. Whenever she revealed a number of these fantasies, she would return to her normal mental state for a few hours; then she would lapse again into another absence, removed again by telling the new fantasies. Clearly, the mental alteration in the absence state was derived from the disturbances accompanying these intensely emotional fantasies.

Subsequently in hypnosis she revealed that her avoidance of drinking from a glass came about after witnessing a dog, which she despised, drinking out of a glass. The dog belonged to her English governess, whom she greatly disliked. After this revelation her symptom disappeared permanently. No one had ever before cured a hysterical symptom through such a "talking cure." Breuer and Freud realized that Anna's symptoms were remnants of earlier, highly emotionally charged experiences determined by memories and feelings from past events.

In another session, she recalled being by her father's sickbed and falling into a reverie. She imagined a snake in the room trying to bite her father and tried to frighten it off by waving her arms, but she found that they could not move. This intensely emotional feeling of paralysis initiated her long-term active paralysis and numbness. When this scene was relived in hypnosis, the paralysis ended, the patient was cured, and the treatment was complete.

Freud concluded from the case of Anna and others that such patients suffer from reminiscences and that their symptoms are memory symbols of earlier traumatic events. In addition, according to Freud, mental suppression of such traumatic events means that these emotions are pent up and retained. These imprisoned emotions are then *changed* ("invented") into abnormal physical symptoms and behaviors, giving rise to the multiple symptoms in the illness of "hysteria" (named for the "wandering uterus" thought by the ancient Greeks to cause such multiple symptoms). Breuer and Freud chose the term *hysterical conversion neurosis* for this displacement process. These patients were entirely unaware of the symbolic connection of their symptoms to the traumatic events. Freud postulated that these memories and their attendant emotions exist out of awareness in the unconscious mind in the illness of "neurosis."

Freud eventually found that he could not hypnotize all his patients, and he began to make the "talking cure" independent of hypnosis. The abandonment of hypnosis presented a formidable difficulty, since the object of treatment was to discover something that neither the doctor nor the patient knew. These memories were imprisoned in the unconscious by a force that Freud felt had to be overcome to bring these repressed thoughts to awareness. To accomplish this, mental resistances had to be overcome along the way.

Freud and his colleagues began to develop other techniques to uncover unconscious conflicts and wishes and to make them available to the patient. He recognized that often the symptoms themselves were indirect, symbolic expressions of the conflict, and that the conflicted emotional reaction was often displaced from the unconscious problem to the symptom. Similarly, he found that the mechanism of repression out of conscious awareness was only partially successful, so that remnants of the underlying problem often surfaced to find expression in indirect yet decipherable ways. Because of the incomplete nature of repression, Freud believed that the individual's mental productions and ideas must reflect the unconscious conflict, and he focused on particular mechanisms to uncover it.

After hypnosis, the technique of *free association* was adopted, wherein the patient would say anything and everything that entered his or her mind, being careful not to censor anything, no matter how irrelevant it might seem. These spontaneous verbal productions are then "psychoanalyzed" so that the analyst is able to discern the relationship of the symptoms to the underlying problem or unconscious conflict. Another technique used in psychoanalysis is the *interpretation of dreams*. Freud recognized that dreams, far from being irrational, unexplainable phenomena, often contain the keys to understanding unconscious mental conflicts and wishes. These unconscious thoughts are defensively acted upon and shaped in characteristic ways to produce what the person remembers as his or her dream. Defense mechanisms commonly seen in dream alteration are symbolization, condensation, and displacement. The actual underlying wish or conflict is indirectly or symbolically represented, or the wish is displaced, i.e., fulfilled or represented in another manner. Condensation is most readily observed in time relationships: childhood events or characters are juxtaposed with later life events or persons.

Clearly, this description is not meant to be anything more than a brief synopsis of dream interpretation in the psychoanalytic sense. For those readers who might be interested in more detail, we suggest Freud's classic book *The Interpretation of Dreams* (1953).

Still another "road to the unconscious" is seen in various bungled acts or mistakes. Freud perceived that common mistakes may have psychological determinants. He especially noted temporary forgetfulness, "slips of the tongue," mistakes in reading and writing, loss or breakage of objects, and other "mishaps." All these events may be provoked by hidden desires, wishes, fears, or other emotions and thus lend themselves to psychoanalytic interpretation.

All of these Freudian concepts have achieved widespread acceptance, or at least popularity, since the time of their introduction. Other Freudian theories, while widely known and studied, are more controversial in terms of their validity or applicability to clinical situations. Among these are Freud's theories of early sexuality. Simply stated, Freud noted that human beings are creatures with a sexual instinct, or libido, and that this instinct finds expression normally in all ages of human development, not just after puberty. Freud believed that these sexual drives are focused and channeled differently at various ages, and that neurotic conflicts seen in adulthood often have their roots in problems in early sexual development. Thus, in early infancy, the baby is seen investing the sexual instinct in an *oral* way through sucking and biting. Too much or too little gratification for these activities is hypothesized to create "oral-dependent" or "oral-aggressive" personality types with resultant neurotic conflicts. Soon the infant passes to a more assertive stage and becomes emotionally interested in bowel training activities. Thus, sexual instincts are channeled into "anal-retentive" and "anal-aggressive" modes of behavior, for example, resisting or giving in to parental demands.

The next stage is discovering one's own genitals, with resulting exploration, touching, or masturbating. This so-called *phallic* stage occurs around ages four to five and seems more relevant to boys than girls. Indeed, the female counterpart, the stage of "penis envy" when little girls discover the absence of external sex organs, has been roundly criticized as blatantly sexist.

It is at ages four to five that so-called *oedipal conflicts* arise, that is, preference by the child for the parent of the opposite sex. This stage may be mild, with only a few fantasies, or it may be quite severe, with aggression and temper tantrums directed toward the parent of the same sex. Freud believed that this oedipal conflict was the basic complex behind virtually every neurosis. In the grade school years, these sexual impulses are quieted, and mental forces such as shame, morality, and disgust are imposed to keep these instincts in restraint. The child is in the latency phase of sexual development, which ends with the dawn of puberty and the focusing of sexual interest on the love object with the goal of reproductive sexuality in the phase of *genital primacy.*

In this normal process, the natural progression can be inhibited or delayed, or the individual can become fixated at an immature level. Under stress, regression can move the person backward developmentally to a more immature stage.

In 1911, Freud described two basic principles that guide mental processes. Both of these principles, the *pleasure principle* and the *reality principle,* are needed to maintain a state of equilibrium in the personality. The pleasure principle refers to the need to avoid pain and seek pleasure through activities which provide immediate gratification directly or which relieve tension. Eventually, the constant pursuit of pleasure and tension relief must give way to dominance by the reality principle, which embodies the demands of external reality. This principle requires *delay* of immediate pleasure or gratification so that pleasure can be achieved in the *long run.* The reality principle, or the delay of immediate gratification, was seen by Freud as a learned or socially conditioned function, and as a feature of emotional maturity and health.

The terms *id, ego,* and *superego* were also coined by Freud to describe particular modes of functioning in the human mind. These terms are not associated with particular brain structures, but with mental functions. Freud conceptualized the id as the repository of instinctual strivings. Sexual, aggressive, and even death instincts were theorized as id-related mental processes. The id is governed by the pleasure principle, which is charged with seeking gratification for its various instinctual cravings.

The superego, according to Freud, comes into being during the transition beyond the oedipal complex. Over the years, superego has come to be almost synonymous with the voice of conscience, the repository of learned social, moral, and religious values inculcated by society. These superego prohibitions put limits on the constant striving impulses of the id and provide reasonable self-control and appropriate socialization for the individual.

The ego consists of mental functions concerned with data processing, memory, calculation, and defense mechanisms. The ego maintains the relationship of the organism to the external world and provides a sense of reality. Ego regulates and modulates instinctual drives by constant application of the reality principle. Ego functions also include characteristic defense mechanisms which control anxiety, preserve self-esteem, and mobilize the energies of the organism toward the satisfaction of various needs. For a thorough discussion of the ego defense mechanisms, we refer the reader to *The Ego and Mechanisms of Defense* by Freud's daughter, Anna Freud (1966). Among the more commonly seen defense mechanisms are the following:

- *Repression* remains the core of most of the defense functions of the ego; it serves to banish from consciousness unpleasant thoughts, ideas, wishes, or attitudes that might be inconsistent with one's ideals or self-concept.
- *Rationalization* consists of making excuses or alibis for instinctual or pleasure-seeking behavior. For example, a compulsive drinker may rationalize his or her excessive alcohol consumption on the basis of the need to relax, unwind, or deal with a tension-producing job or other problem.

- *Denial* is often blatant in psychiatric disturbances. A person may refuse to see the extent of her or his problems or may deny the long-term consequences of her or his acts. Another form of denial is unwillingness to concede the need for help. For example, a compulsive gambler may deny that she or he has a serious problem and refuse a referral to Gamblers Anonymous.
- *Projection* is often seen in paranoid disturbances in which the patient's own unconscious motivation may be "projected" and attributed to others. For example, accusations of infidelity by one's spouse may be a projected jealousy or wish. ("She must be cheating on me. I would if I could.") More commonly seen is *projection of blame.* It serves defensively to exonerate the person from self-blame or social disapproval. "He made me do it" or "It's his fault, not mine" are commonly occurring human responses indicating a degree of projection of blame.
- *Sublimation* is one of the healthier defense mechanisms. It allows the ego to channel instinctually determined energies into socially adaptive and constructive outlets, for example, becoming a soldier in order to sublimate powerful aggressive urges in a socially appropriate way.
- *Compensation* is another healthy defense mechanism that allows an individual to maintain self-esteem in the face of certain shortcomings by investing energies in another, gratification-producing area. The painfully shy, socially introverted young boy who becomes an outstanding scholar and earns a good deal of self-respect and social approval is a good example of compensation.

As a final contribution, Freud noted the phenomenon of *transference,* in which the patient displays seemingly inappropriate emotions toward the doctor or therapist; such emotions are said to be neurotically (and unconsciously) transferred from their earlier objects and now find expression in the doctor-patient relationship. Analysis of the patient's transference reactions is often a keystone of psychoanalytic work. The therapist will usually go to great lengths to avoid influencing the transference; often the therapist presents a rather bland facade to the patient or even sits out of the patient's view, saying little. Such techniques are stressful yet still commonly used in psychoanalysis. The patient responds to the bland therapist's facade by inserting his or her own transference reactions, revealing hidden thoughts and emotions.

This process of overcoming resistance and uncovering the unconscious wishes or conflicts of the patient is the essential basis of psychoanalysis. Viewed in a psychoanalytic light, the repressed wish or forbidden conflict is reexamined and placed in a newer, more mature, detached perspective. The repressed conflict is understood as normal and is reconciled with the person's forbidding conscience (superego), or it is redirected into other channels to serve the person in better ways (sublimation). Conscious thought and mature adult choices now prevail where only unconscious emotion and unexplained symptoms formerly dominated.

MODERN PSYCHIATRIC TREATMENT

We hasten to add that the terms *psychoanalysis, psychiatry,* and *psychotherapy* are not all synonymous, yet they are often confused by the public. We have spoken now at length about theories underlying psychoanalysis, yet this is just one theory and branch of psychiatric practice. *Most psychiatrists are not psychoanalysts* and do not necessarily use the techniques of free association and analysis of dreams or "slips" on a constant basis. Orthodox psychoanalysis is a discipline unto itself, requiring enrollment in a psychoanalytic institute for several years. The enrollee, usually a trained psychiatrist or psychologist, must train as an analyst under supervision and participate in and pay for his or her own personal analysis. Certified psychoanalysts are generally located in large cities on the Eastern seaboard. Psychoanalysis (as opposed to psychotherapy) as a treatment can be very expensive. Psychoanalytic candidates are seen four to five times per week in one-hour sessions, often for several years. The expense of this, plus the inability of the analyst to see large numbers of patients, makes this modality vulnerable to the criticism that it is too costly or impractical for general use. Yet in spite of its waning influence, psychoanalysis has left its mark on psychiatry, and "brief psychoanalytically oriented psychotherapy" is now widely available to most patients at moderate cost. Most patients now see their therapists once a week or less often, usually for a few months or longer, depending on the severity of the illness.

In addition to psychoanalytically oriented psychotherapy, the patient (and the referring clergyperson) are now confronted with a sizeable array of newer, more practical therapies. Among these are Gestalt therapy, rational emotive therapy, reality therapy, and transactional analysis. These therapies tend to focus on the patient's *current* situation and feelings as manifestations of a lifelong style of behavior that may be problematic. By acquiring awareness of these lifelong patterns, one can begin a process of changing them. Often such therapies are done in groups. At times, these therapies can appear "confrontational," but usually it is the patient's maladaptive thinking, attitudes, behaviors, and emotions that are being confronted, not the patient. Problem-oriented psychotherapy has an even more "here-and-now" focus on immediate problems in a practical way.

Another significant development has been the evolution of family therapy, in which the identified patient is the entire family system, rather than a single individual. Typically, stresses are identified and resolved, communication is opened up, and negative reactions and behaviors are replaced with positive responses. Family therapy is particularly useful in cases of disturbed family dynamics, such as are often found with symptomatic children and adolescents.

Practitioners of these forms of psychotherapy need not necessarily be psychiatrists or MDs. Many competent psychotherapists are found in the ranks of psychologists, social workers, and other mental health professionals. In general, these psychotherapeutic modalities are better suited to emotional disorders of lesser severity, e.g., situational reactions, milder depressions, and anxiety states. More severe emotional disorders, such as those involving loss of contact with reality, severe disruption of functional ability, and possible danger to self or others, require the intervention of a trained psychiatrist, who has in his or her therapeutic armamentarium psychiatric medications, hospitalization, and even electroconvulsive therapy, if needed.

In order for the pastor to find his or her place on the health care team, he or she must have some understanding of these treatment modalities. "Talking cures" or psychotherapies have their limitations and may even be antitherapeutic at times; for example, some uncovering or emotive therapies might produce violent reactions with paranoid psychotics. Although Freud revolutionized our understanding of the mind and mental processes in milder forms of mental illness (neuroses), he recognized that psychoanalysis probably could do little to alter the more severe illnesses, or psychoses.

In fact, little could be done for severely ill mental patients until 1935, when von Meduna began treating psychotics with camphor-induced convulsions. This treatment was based on clinical observations that psychotics became less symptomatic after a seizure, and also on observations (later proven) of a low incidence of severe mental illness in epileptics. Soon, Cerletti and Bini discovered that convulsions could be induced much more reliably by a modest electric current passing briefly through the brain. Electroconvulsive therapy (ECT), or "shock therapy," eventually became widely used for many types of psychiatric disorders. Regrettably, ECT has received tremendous negative publicity as "barbaric" treatment. Critics of ECT claim the treatment has been overused and can be followed by a degree of brain damage. Such publicity has obscured the inescapable and widely held conclusion that ECT, at our present state of knowledge, remains the safest, fastest, least expensive, and most effective treatment for *some* severely ill patients. In other words, reputable psychiatrists and mental hospitals do use ECT, but they use it sparingly and only for certain conditions. Certainly, as with any medical procedure, the potential exists for indiscriminate use and abuse, and "shock mills" are to be avoided.

What happens when a patient receives ECT? He or she is usually put to sleep under short-acting general anesthesia; then his or her muscles are immobilized with a drug to prevent movement during the seizure. A brief (one-half second) shock is administered to the head and imitates a typical grand-mal seizure lasting a minute or so. When the seizure subsides, the anesthetist supports the patient with assisted respiration until breathing begins spontaneously in another minute or so. The entire procedure may take less than ten minutes. These treatments are often given three to five times per week, and a total of between five and twenty treatments may be needed for severe illness.

Some confusion and memory impairment after treatment are to be expected, but these usually clear spontaneously in a few days. Long-term brain impairment has been alleged in some cases involving many treatments, but these assertions are still controversial. For the present, ECT remains a safe, effective treatment for specific conditions, especially severe psychotic depressive reactions in the elderly. Often the treatment is lifesaving.

Hospital care is usually indicated, at least initially, in the treatment of severe illness. Most often, hospitalization consists of environmental supervision and support with a system of increasing "privileges," allowing more autonomy as the patient improves. Many psychiatric hospital units have a locked door on the ward to prevent confused patients from wandering off. Most of the stable, well-oriented patients will have "passes" allowing them to leave the ward to visit family or go for walks. Most hospital units provide group and individual therapy, medications, or ECT, if needed, as well as a variety of "activity therapies," such as art therapy, dance therapy, creative therapy, or vocational rehabilitation. Some units have special programs for alcoholics, drug dependents, or others. Most psychiatrists will hospitalize patients exhibiting loss of contact with reality, disorientation, or danger to self or others.

Psychiatric or psychotropic medications are now widely and routinely used for severe emotional disorders and for many of the milder ones. They should be prescribed and monitored regularly by a knowledgeable psychiatrist, since their use is often a complicated matter. At the moment, medications are the treatment of choice for most patients with severe emotional illness. Most of the severely ill will require fairly high doses in the acute illness phase, then lower maintenance doses to prevent relapses and further episodes. These modern medicines have truly revolutionized the care of the emotionally ill and have been the single most important factor in the dramatic census decline in long-term psychiatric hospitals in recent years.

Psychiatrists use several classes of psychotropic medications, including the following:

- *Major tranquilizers, antipsychotics, or neuroleptics.* These agents are used for severe agitation, confusion, and thinking disorders characteristic of the severe psychoses. Examples are Thorazine, Stelazine, Haldol, Clozaril, Risperdal, and Zyprexa. They will often be used in high doses for acute mania, acute schizophrenic reactions, and agitated "organic" brain disorders. Tolerance (the need to increase dosages) does not develop, and these medications are nonaddicting. Side effects can include drowsiness, stiffness, blurred vision, low blood pressure, and fainting. White blood cells must be monitored with Clozaril. Muscle stiffness can be countered with another medication such as Cogentin or

Benadryl. Each medication has unique side effects and indications for its use. Treatment must therefore be individualized by the psychiatrist.

- *Minor tranquilizers or anxiolytics.* These agents are useful for the temporary management of anxiety states, insomnia, heart palpitations, and other physical problems caused by excessive nervousness. Examples are Librium, Valium, Serax, Ativan, and Xanax. These agents carry some risk of inducing medication dependence and addiction. Side effects include sedation and alcohol potentiation. They are generally used on a short-term basis, and they should be used only with great caution (or not at all) in people with a history of addiction to alcohol or drugs.

- *Antidepressants.* These agents are useful in the treatment of all but the mildest of depressive disorders. Although not very useful for mild "reactive" or "situational" depressions (which usually resolve spontaneously), they are indicated for long-term depressive states of medium to serious severity. There are now many classes and types of antidepressants in use, but a comprehensive review of these is beyond the scope of this book. Two major groups of antidepressants predominate, however. The so-called tricyclic antidepressants (TCAs) have been in use since the 1950s and include such medications as Elavil and Tofranil. Common side effects of tricyclics are weight gain, drowsiness, or drop in blood pressure. Although nonaddicting, they can be dangerous in overdose. Because of these undesirable side effects and lethal overdose potential, another class of antidepressants is the preferred initial treatment for depression—the SSRIs. These drugs, the selective serotonin reuptake inhibitors, include Prozac, Paxil, Zoloft, Serzone, and many others. Some newer drugs seem to combine the effects of the TCAs and SSRIs in a broad spectrum medication. All of these drugs work by improving and speeding up brain-cell activity, by stimulating one or more chemical reactions in and between the cells. The SSRIs have fewer side effects (decreased sexual interest and orgasmic delay are frequently seen), and are nonlethal in an overdose.

- *Mood stabilizers.* Lithium carbonate is in this class and is extremely effective for bipolar illness, a cyclical illness of great severity with pronounced mood highs and lows, or fluctuations. Lithium often works extremely well in preventing relapses. Un-

fortunately, blood levels of the drug must be frequently monitored to avoid toxic buildup, which can be dangerous. Side effects
can include thyroid suppression, drowsiness, confusion, and
nausea. Lithium can be dangerous if taken in an overdose. It is
not addicting. Other mood stabilizers include drugs used to prevent convulsions, such as Tegretol, Neurontin, or Topamax.
They are usually well tolerated, do not cause addiction, and
have few side effects. All of these mood stabilizers decrease irritability and prevent violent mood swings, especially in manic or
bipolar depressions with pronounced highs and lows or marked
irritability and impulsivity.

Very often the minister will find emotionally disturbed patients on
prescribed medication under the care of a physician. Many patients
do not like to take these medications, and some have no awareness of
their need for taking them. It is important to realize that the decision
to place a patient on medicine *or to take her or him off medicine* is a
medical decision, and should be made only by a physician, not by the
patient or by a non-medical professional such as a clergyperson.
Most patients deteriorate when medication is discontinued. Clergy
should avoid the mistake of making medical decisions when this is
not within their expertise. The best policy is to support the physician's
recommendations and encourage the patient to follow instructions
carefully and completely. If the patient is having trouble with the
medications, the best policy is for both patient and clergy to contact
the physician, or to get a second psychiatric opinion if questions remain.

In summary, clergy who aspire to work with mentally ill people as
part of a healing team will soon realize that psychiatry is not a "one
size fits all" proposition. Scarcely two people are alike in their symptoms, illnesses, and response to different treatments. Most severely ill
patients will be offered medications, hospitalization or intensive outpatient treatment, and some form (or several forms) of psychotherapy. Family involvement is usually encouraged, but often the family
(if any remains) does not wish to participate. Activity therapies, such
as various forms of crafts and physical therapy, are used as evaluative
tools to assess progress, and also as restorative aids in the return to
normal routines of life. The most severely ill may require multiple

medications, close supervision, protective housing, or electroconvulsive therapy.

The pastoral counselor should endeavor first to understand the nature of the person's illness and the problematic signs, symptoms, and behaviors the staff is trying to treat. The pastor should then become aware of the treatment plan, at least in a general way (e.g., medications, psychotherapy, hospitalization), and only then should the pastor ask, "What can I do to provide counsel, enlightenment, hope, support, or a spiritual intervention *that is consistent with* the specific needs of this patient and with the treatment plan of the professional staff?" If the pastor truly operates in this way, basing his or her ministrations on the *specific needs* of the patient and the specific plans of the staff, he or she can provide wonderfully meaningful and perhaps life-changing pastoral interventions. These pastoral works can take many forms, including scriptural guidance, sacramental services, and restorative pastoral counseling. Using these and other spiritual tools in a highly specific way for each individual patient, the pastoral counselor will see that he or she can quickly become an accepted, valued agent of change in the recovery process.

The recovery process is seldom instantaneous; it is normally a prolonged struggle to find healthier thinking, attitudes, emotions, and behaviors. In treatment, the search for the better way is aided and guided by many helpers or links in the chain of recovery. Each link contributes a small but important share. The pastor should remember this analogy and work diligently to see that his or her link is strongly, knowledgeably, and responsibly forged.

Chapter 2

The Depressed Person

OVERVIEW

Depression of mood is a syndrome of emotional distress, often precipitated by a traumatic event, which overwhelms the vulnerable person and produces a variety of characteristic symptoms. Depressions may range in severity from mild, short-term moodiness to full-blown loss of contact with reality with suicidal or homicidal potential. Depressive disorders are among the most common problems seen by psychiatrists and pastoral counselors and are also, fortunately, among the problems that are easiest to treat successfully. The following cases are presented to demonstrate some fairly typical situations that pastoral counselors are likely to see.

CASE EXAMPLES

Mary

Mary is the wife of a prominent executive in your parish. Now, at the age of fifty-five, she advises you that she is seeing a psychiatrist for repeated crying spells. You are surprised at her appearance. Ordinarily she is very well groomed, but her makeup, hairdo, and clothing are not up to her usual impeccable standard. She appears sad and has little to say. She complains of loss of interest in life and general feelings of worthlessness. She has lost all interest in sex and says that she would not blame her husband if he found a girlfriend. She attributes most of her problems to "menopause," but on further questioning she notes that six months ago her last remaining child went off to college in a distant state. Her husband is away on business trips often, so she has been spending most of her days in a large suburban home by herself with little to do. She has been eating more lately, mostly out of boredom, and she has gained a substantial amount of weight. This too is quite distressing. She has just begun seeing a psychiatrist at the urging of her husband.

Catherine

Catherine comes to see you because she says she has been having problems sleeping at night. She has many bad dreams, and most of these have to do with her parents. Catherine's aged parents were both living with her until about two years ago, when her mother died of diabetic complications. Catherine had been extremely involved in her care until she died. Catherine's father lived on, but gradually became demented to the point that he was unable to feed himself or handle his toilet needs. He did not recognize members of the family, and on two occasions he was found wandering around naked in the neighborhood. Catherine endured all of these difficulties for two years and only recently forced herself to place her father in a nursing home. His emotional reaction to this experience was very negative, and, in an agitated state, he fell down the stairs of the nursing home and broke his hip. An infection set in, and he died a few days later. Catherine relates that she has frequent crying spells and is constantly preoccupied with thoughts of her parents. She feels that she has let them down and was directly responsible for their deaths. She now finds that her obsessions about this are so unrelenting that she is unable to keep up with her normal activities, and her family is becoming very concerned about her. She has no appetite and has lost twenty pounds in the past few months.

Patricia

Patricia, a forty-seven-year-old woman in your parish, comes to see you about a "marital problem." She states that three months ago, after twenty-five years of marriage, her husband left her and moved in with his young secretary. Patricia still lives in the family home with their two teenage children. Her husband is providing her with some support and has made repeated requests for a divorce. She is so far refusing to grant it on "religious grounds," in spite of her friends' advice to divorce him. Patricia has been spending a great deal of money on various kinds of medical treatment. She is suffering from severe backache, which began about the time her husband left. She has been taking various pain medications and tranquilizers, but she does not seem to be getting much more than temporary relief. She says she feels helpless and outraged at her circumstances, but also notes that she has never been very assertive and that she has always placed a premium on being a good and forgiving person. She does not blame her husband for leaving her; she feels that she should have done more to meet his needs and be a better spouse to him. She discovered yesterday, however, that her husband had apparently withdrawn money they both had been saving for the children's college education to pay for an expensive ocean cruise with his new girlfriend. Patricia says she feels helpless and immobilized and does not know what to do. She has an attorney, but he is also representing her husband. She has not sought out her own separate counsel because she did not want to spend the extra money.

Vince

Vince is a thirty-two-year-old male who comes to see you because he is unhappy about his personal life. He is fed up with himself and feels that it is impossible for him to maintain a long-term relationship with anyone. He feels unlovable and cannot see why anyone would be interested in him. He starts to sob violently in your office, advises you that three weeks ago his wife of one year left him, and says that he just received divorce papers this morning. Until he married his wife, Vince had been living with his mother. He and his mother were abandoned by Vince's father when he was two years old. As a result, he never knew his father and had to become "the man of the house" at a very early age. He and his mother were left in bad shape financially by the desertion, and from age ten Vince worked in various odd jobs to help pay household expenses. Two years ago, Vince's mother died of cancer, and he began serious dating for the first time in his life. He met a twenty-year-old woman at a church function and married her after a courtship of six weeks. Soon after the marriage, Vince became extremely jealous and was unable to let his wife out of his sight. He would call repeatedly at work to check up on her. He would frequently go through her clothing and personal effects to check for notes or other evidence from possible suitors. He could not believe that he was a worthwhile mate, and he would constantly belittle himself in comparison to others. If his wife watched a television show, he would become morose and despondent if the show featured a handsome male. After months of paranoid jealousy, unprovoked by his wife, he was given an ultimatum to seek psychiatric help "or else." He did not obtain psychiatric help because he felt he was not "that bad yet." Now that he has received divorce papers, he is extremely despondent and has even talked of committing suicide by carbon monoxide poisoning.

Jim

Jim is a twenty-year-old junior at a nearby college who was brought in by his parents because of recent personality changes and fear that he would commit suicide. His parents say he was a "model child" who followed in his older brother's footsteps until about eighteen months ago. His older brother has recently graduated from medical school and is continuing his training at a prestigious hospital. The patient's father is a physician also, and Jim says that it has long been his parents' goal to see both their sons become doctors. Jim says that this was his goal too. However, in the last year or so he has had increasingly serious problems with the premedical curriculum. His grades have not been good, and he has become depressed and preoccupied with them. He has lost interest in school in the past few months and has recently missed classes for weeks at a time. The school counselor contacted his parents, advising them that their son was doing poorly and that he was perhaps having a breakdown of some kind. Lately he has been religiously preoccupied and has spent a good deal of time with some religious groups on campus. His parents noticed that he has been more morose, sullen, quiet, and withdrawn in the past few months. Recently, his parents came across some poetry he had written that appeared to be emphasizing suicide as a solution to one's problems. His parents have become increasingly alarmed and feel their son needs help.

Amy

Amy is a sixty-seven-year-old woman who was apparently a successful grade-school teacher until her retirement two years ago. Ordinarily quite fastidious and vivacious in nature, she is now letting everything go, including grooming, household responsibilities, and personal affairs. Her husband reports that she merely paces around the house all day, constantly worrying about her health. She is morbidly obsessed with having cancer, and although she has had several recent checkups, she has not been reassured by the doctor's claim that nothing is wrong. She feels that she is about to die soon from cancer, and that no one will tell her the "truth" about her impending death. Lately she has taken to staying in bed, constantly complaining about pains which seem to shift from her abdomen to her head. Her husband was recently surprised to learn from her that she feels insects are gnawing at her brain. She has refused to see a psychiatrist but has agreed to talk with you, her minister. When you see her, she is tearful, agitated, and overwhelmingly preoccupied with the certainty of her fatal disease. In fact, she cuts the session short because she has to go home and "get her affairs in order" so she can die with everything in place.

Connie

Connie is a forty-five-year-old woman who appears to have been entirely well until approximately one year ago. Her husband comes with her to see you in your office and states that she has had a marked personality change since that time. For no apparent reason, Connie began to be morbidly preoccupied with the health of her family members. She feels that whenever they are out of her sight, they have been killed in a traffic accident or are ill and being rushed to the emergency room. When the family members return, she is only temporarily reassured. As soon as they are out of sight again, she begins to have the obsessions once more. Also, her husband reports other changes in her thinking. She is now obsessed that someone has bugged the house and the telephone line. She does not know who this is, or why it would be so, but she refuses to discuss anything further within the home. She takes family members outside to walk around the block to discuss anything, lest they be overheard by the "bugs." She refuses to talk on the telephone because she feels that it is tapped. When you ask her why, she reports that she has been under surveillance by foreign spies, and that she and her family are objects of a clandestine plot. She feels certain that she and her family will be poisoned or killed as part of this conspiratorial plot. She has become so obsessed with these ruminations that she is no longer functioning at home. She constantly calls her husband and other family members when they are out to ascertain whether they are well. She has frequent terrible crying spells if she is unable to reach a family member for more than a few minutes. When you ask her what she thinks about all this, she replies that she is deeply afraid that she is perhaps going insane, because in her better moments she knows that these things cannot possibly be true. Yet when left to herself, she returns to the same morbid preoccupations.

RECOGNITION

People with significant depression will usually complain of fatigue, apathy, listlessness, and lack of energy. They often lose interest in personal grooming, hygiene, and household responsibilities. Morbid preoccupation with problems may occur, and the person may also demonstrate feelings of hopelessness and worthlessness. Self-destructive attitudes may be present, ranging in severity from merely giving up, or lack of concern about death, to overt self-destructiveness and suicidal intent. Very often, so-called vegetative signs of depression will be present. These include impaired sleep, loss of appetite, weight loss, loss of sexual interest, suppression of normal menstrual periods, and actual inhibition of motion. Sleep impairment may be manifested by early morning awakening, nightmares with depressive themes, or trouble falling asleep. Appetite may be suppressed or increased out of boredom and apathy. Weight loss or weight gain may occur, as well as constipation. Crying spells may be frequent or nonexistent. Depression may, in fact, be masked by physical symptoms and numerous medical complaints.

ASSESSMENT OF SEVERITY

Assessment of severity is a more complicated matter than recognition. There is tremendous individual variability in susceptibility to depression. Some people never experience depressed emotions. Others become depressed with relatively little provocation. The following questions need to be answered when assessing the severity of a depressive reaction.

1. Is reality testing preserved? In other words, does the person have full contact with reality, and is judgment reasonably sound? If not, this indicates a psychotic degree of depression and, in all likelihood, psychiatric help is going to be needed immediately.
2. Is there much danger of homicide or suicide? When assessing patients with serious degrees of depression, probe for suicidal thinking. The inexperienced pastoral counselor will be surprised to see how many people have given serious thought to suicide at one time or another in their lives. Suicidal rumination

or preoccupation, or the presence of a plan or the means of carrying it out, should always be taken seriously. A serious possibility of suicide or homicidal loss of control should immediately be referred to the psychiatrist or suicide prevention agency or to the emergency room. People who are seriously contemplating suicide will usually require psychiatric hospitalization until stability returns.

3. Are vegetative signs of depression present? These signs are manifestations of secondary physical reactions to prolonged depression, and include loss of appetite, weight loss, sleep changes, apathy, impairment of motion, and sexual or menstrual suppression. The presence of a significant number of these organic manifestations of depression heralds a more serious problem, one that will usually require psychiatric intervention, possibly with medication.

4. What is the level of discomfort or suffering experienced by the person or his or her family? Obviously, the greater the degree of subjective distress, the more serious the depression is likely to be. However, subjective distress is not always present, and the person may be merely giving up and may even feel that he or she deserves to be punished. Often one needs to look at the general level of overall functioning and the presence of personality change or deterioration from a normal state. Clearly, it is very difficult to assess the extent of a depressive episode unless one has a reasonable idea of the person's level of functioning prior to the depressive attack. Dramatic changes always are to be taken more seriously.

5. Has the person had previous professional treatment for a depressive episode? Previous treatment with psychiatric hospitalization, high-dose medications, or shock treatment should always alert the pastoral counselor to the presence of a serious difficulty.

CRISIS INTERVENTION

Depending on the severity of the depression, crisis intervention may take many forms. With more serious depressive disorders characterized by loss of contact with reality, suicidal intent, vegetative signs, subjective suffering, and a history of previous treatment, referral for psychiatric evaluation is always indicated. The majority of patients with any of these symptoms will probably require psychiatric hospitalization for the initial phases of treatment. In the psychiatric hospital, it is likely that the psychiatrist will attempt a combination of antidepressant medication, psychotherapy, and various activity therapies. Making a referral to the psychiatrist or hospital may be difficult. Most people have a tendency to avoid doctors and psychiatrists, and there may be concern about the stigmatizing effects of a psychiatric hospitalization. Nonetheless, you should assist the person in any way possible in making this initial contact for evaluation.

It is a good idea to call the psychiatrist's office, emergency room, or hospital directly from your office with the person present. Offering to accompany the person to the psychiatric evaluation is even more supportive. In any case, it is best to avoid a situation wherein the person faces a psychiatric evaluation alone. If the psychiatrist recommends hospitalization, it is generally best to support this view and help the patient accept it. Most will be concerned about appearances, finances, fear of the unknown, stigma, or inability to give up daily responsibilities. The best response to patient resistance is to point out that the goal is to get well first. Advise the patient that you are not abandoning him or her in the psychiatric hospital. Rather, you are offering continued assistance and will visit or call on a frequent basis to offer support, counseling, encouragement, and spiritual guidance. Make this offer to both the psychiatrist and the patient, and you will seldom be rebuffed.

It is strongly advisable for the pastoral counselor to visit the patient in the hospital. Often people are more depressed immediately after hospitalization. The first few days may be very rough, often with tremendous emotional turmoil due to self-blaming or sense of failure. The pastoral counselor can help these first few days go more smoothly and less painfully for the suffering person. Pastoral counseling in a hospital setting should be positive and supportive. It should be supportive of the suggestions of the doctor and staff, and if the minister finds it difficult to support their views, he or she should speak directly with the treating physician, rather than share his or her views with the patient. If the patient has lost contact with reality, sympathetic but reality-oriented conversation is the rule. The minister should not be too coercive or insistent, but instead factual and relaxed. Mistaken ideas or delusional thinking are best called into question rather than openly and directly challenged, unless the patient tolerates such directness well. If suicidal ideation is present, spiritual counseling can be extremely valuable if it emphasizes God's love, forgiveness, patience, and concern for the suffering patient. Additional themes to emphasize are personal self-worth, healthy self-assertion, and attitudes of serenity and gratitude. "Counting one's blessings," often on paper, is a useful exercise to distract from negative ruminations.

The pastor will find that in general family members are distraught and unsettled about the patient's illness, and that usually the family equilibrium is terribly disrupted. Since most doctors do not have adequate time to deal with family members during a psychiatric hospitalization, the minister should be in contact with the family and provide sympathetic and optimistic support. If communication between the doctor and the family appears to be poor, the minister can perhaps facilitate better dialogue.

COUNSELING IN THE RECOVERY PHASE

After hospital discharge or, conversely, if outpatient management alone is sufficient, follow-up pastoral counseling can be of great benefit. If the patient remains on a regimen of medication and professional counseling sessions, these should be strongly endorsed, and she or he should be encouraged to follow physician recommendations in these matters very carefully. If it appears that the patient has difficulty with compliance, or if physician instructions are not well understood, contact the physician directly to ask for an explanation or to offer additional pastoral assistance.

Assuming these matters are in order, what should pastoral counseling consist of in this phase? As the reader can judge from the case examples given in this chapter, depressed patients vary tremendously in their emotional difficulties and emotional needs. There is no substitute for familiarity with the patient and his or her unique problem, and this is one area in which the minister might have some advantage over other members of the health care team. Perhaps he or she has known the patient for years and may have a clearer idea of how the patient is fitting into his social milieu.

In general, the pastor should be alert for the following depressive themes, illustrated in the previously noted cases:

1. *Losses or grief reactions.* Mary is an example of a woman who appears to have "lost" her children as they have grown up and moved away from her. Once this happened, she may have lost a good deal of her self-respect and even personal identity as a competent mother. Other losses in life may be even more devastating. Loss of one's spouse is, by most professional estimates, the most traumatic event that a person experiences in life. Similarly, the loss of a child can have a grievous and long-lasting depressive impact. Losses are best dealt with through counseling that emphasizes acceptance of the finality of the loss, appropriate (and time-limited) displays of grieving emotion, and surrender to the will of God and Divine Providence. Normal grief reactions or reactions to loss will commonly last for six months to two years. Severe depressive reactions to loss extending beyond that time imply a serious problem. Looking ahead to the future, while making concrete plans for a new life and adjusting to the loss, is helpful. Concrete suggestions by the pastoral counselor and assistance in carrying out the initial steps of a new life are much appreciated. Often the person is paralyzed or immobilized by the loss and resulting psychological trauma, so concrete assistance in getting started fresh is extremely helpful. Practical concerns, such as getting a driver's license, filing for benefits, or taking care of financial responsibilities, are situations in which tangible assistance is invaluable.

2. *Guilt reactions,* such as the one exemplified by Catherine, who placed her father in a nursing home, may be dealt with by inquiring first as to whether the person feels the need for forgiveness or feels the inability to obtain forgiveness. Sometimes, because this need for forgiveness is all out of proportion to the perceived wrongdoing, it may initially be better to deal with the person's own perceived need for forgiveness than to assist him or her in finding realistic forgiveness. It may be helpful to remind him or her that God is all-forgiving, and if He can provide forgiveness, then we should certainly forgive ourselves. Often, however, disproportionate guilt reactions reflect unresolved guilt or problems from the distant past. It may be advisable to go beyond the present guilt reaction to see if there are other things in the past about which the person feels unresolved guilt. Another helpful approach is to counsel an attitude of surrender to Divine Providence and the will of God. What is done is done, and nothing can change it. We have to accept things the way they are and live in the present. Guilt is not a particularly helpful emotion to people who

suffer from excesses of it. It is best to put an end to guilt reactions and move on with life as soon as reasonably possible. Guilt reactions are often terribly difficult to eliminate. People who suffer from excessive guilt are often predisposed toward it by past experience. Because of this built-in conditioned susceptibility, once a guilt-provoking experience occurs it often becomes magnified far out of proportion and seems to trigger an endless cycle of guilt and suffering. Persistence, patience, and time are needed, but professional psychiatric help may well be required to get to the underlying problem.

3. *Retroflexed or self-directed stifled anger* is often a cause of depression seen in people who are overcontrolled and exceptionally accommodating to others. In the case cited, Patricia, abandoned by her husband for another woman, cannot bring herself to take an assertive stance to resolve her marital situation. Her husband even rubs her nose in it by spending their hard-earned money on his girlfriend, yet Patricia is still unable to take any action on her own behalf. Instead, she blames herself. This is not an atypical reaction for people who have difficulty expressing anger or assertiveness or even acting in their own self-interests. It might be helpful to note that Christ Himself demonstrated appropriate anger and took action against the moneychangers in the Temple. At times, acting assertively in one's own self-interest is the only healthy thing to do. In fact, the pathological inability to be assertive or to act in one's self-interest is an open invitation for exploitation by others. Such pathological nonassertiveness appears to have been the case with Patricia. Counseling should emphasize taking charge of one's future while realistically protecting oneself from victimization. Certainly Patricia's self-interest might be served by obtaining her own legal counsel. Once counsel is obtained, following through with the legal process of divorce can be difficult and painful. The pastoral counselor can be of great assistance in offering support and mobilizing energy to deal with this situation, while maintaining a degree of impartiality. Seeking a positive outcome for all involved is a useful pastoral objective. People who suffer from retroflexed anger need to develop a different style of functioning. In general, they tend to be too quiet, long-suffering, patient, and other-directed for their own good. They need more "backbone" and "permission" to be assertive and to meet their needs actively. This is their natural right, and the pastoral counselor should encourage them.

In addition, special courses and reading materials in assertiveness training are often of value.

4. *Early losses in life* sensitize individuals to the prospect of losses later in life and may predispose individuals to later bouts of depression. While this is not always the case, Vince, described in the case examples, may well demonstrate such a problem. Abandoned by his father at an early age, he has unmet dependency needs that cause him to take a clinging, excessively protective posture toward his loved ones. He is so overwhelmed with *anxiety* about the possibility of enduring an additional loss that he drives his loved one away with jealous overprotectiveness. As a result, he blames himself, suffers a grievous depression, and even considers suicide. Vince appears to be troubled with *pathological insecurities,* but one also sees a good deal of *neurotic self-blame* in people who have been abandoned. Very often the child feels, "Daddy left because I was bad. I did something that drove him away." This message, repeated to oneself over the years, gradually erodes self-esteem until the person may come to believe that, in fact, he or she deserved to be abandoned. Ideally, these neurotic past fears and anxieties will be brought to the surface in the context of psychotherapy; if this is not available, ministerial counseling can do much to alter these underlying attitudes. The person needs to reexamine his or her reaction to early childhood loss from a mature, adult perspective. Patients must understand that they had nothing to do with the reason for the abandonment and they must begin to formulate a more positive, accepting attitude toward themselves as worthwhile, loveable human beings. In addition, they must practice new patterns in relationships, such as, in this example, Vince becoming less possessive. People who have experienced abandonment or parental death often have difficulty giving love and affection. Having been disappointed in early loving relationships, they are often unable to risk the emotional vulnerability inherent in loving and closeness. Cultivating new relationships on the basis of trust and openness is a long-term proposition during which the person may need support, encouragement, and strengthening pastoral love. The outlook is often problematic without a long-term effort at attitudinal change.

5. *Losses of self-esteem* are frequent causes of depressive reactions. In Jim's case he has aspired to follow in his father's footsteps to become a physician. The family may have reinforced this goal over the years, and it may appear to the patient that there is no escape from

admitting total failure in this endeavor. His reaction to his school difficulties is one of functional immobilization and escalating problems. The resulting paralysis seems only to make his problems worse. He appears to be groping for some semblance of self-esteem through acceptance by a religious group. This marked degree of personality change may be suggestive of a serious reaction, and professional help should be sought for an evaluation. Family counseling may be advisable since there seems to be such a fixed role expectation for him. Settling on realistic goals and allowing permission for the boy to alter the family's expectations may be required. The family may not even be aware that his is a failure reaction with loss of self-esteem. Openly communicating about these matters while mobilizing family support for the son will initiate the process of healing. Pastoral care should include counseling regarding the worth of every individual, the specialness of each person, and God's divine love for every person. The person should be allowed to maintain his or her own self-worth apart from the necessity of achieving particular goals. It may be helpful to encourage the suffering person to redirect his or her efforts toward healthy satisfactions that are more consistent with his or her own aptitudes and gifts.

6. Finally, the cases of Amy and Connie illustrate depressed patients experiencing serious *loss of contact with reality*. In the first case, the patient was morbidly concerned with the presence of life-threatening disease in her own body. In the second, more global loss of contact with reality was present, with paranoia and fear of disaster for the patient's family members. Both of these patients will initially require intensive psychiatric treatment, but in the postacute phase they will be in much better contact with reality, and the pastoral care methods discussed previously can be utilized. Most often, such patients will be placed on long-term maintenance medications and will need encouragement to continue following the doctor's instructions. Any tendency to relapse into obsessive, depressive delusions should be pointed out and discouraged. Often, a policy of kind encouragement, support, and loving pastoral ministry is all that is required. Sometimes, however, the delusional content will change and appear in another form, such as self-blame, suicidal preoccupation, or new paranoid ideas. Should these appear, the pastor should help the patient inform the psychiatrist so that the situation can be quickly reevaluated. Counseling should be reality oriented in a sympathetic

way. Self-reproach should be discouraged, and persistent irrational obsessions should be gently brushed aside. It is usually best to focus on future plans and specifics. For further discussion of reality impairment, see Chapter 6.

Chapter 3

The Anxious Person

OVERVIEW

Anxiety is a nonspecific emotion that may be produced by worry, fear, tension, or conflict. In mild degree, anxiety is not necessarily pathological. Rather, anxiety can be considered the body's normal warning signal in response to situations or reactions that are distressing or dangerous. Once anxiety is felt, it mobilizes the person to employ defensive reactions, such as "fight-or-flight" maneuvers, that overcome or avoid the feared object or situation. However, this useful and perhaps lifesaving function of anxiety may be subject to changes in expression that render it a problem. Primitive solutions such as fight or flight may not be permissible or practical in a complex, interwoven societal situation. The cause of stress may be a continuous one, such as a job or family member. But the stress can also be internal, as in a conditioned, overreactive tension response to normal environmental stimuli. All people experience anxiety to a greater or lesser degree, and the causes of anxiety are variable among people. Since anxiety is a normal emotion, reactive to normal and abnormal life stresses, we all must develop coping skills and adaptive psychological and behavioral mechanisms for managing anxiety in a healthy way. When these normal coping skills or adaptive mechanisms are overwhelmed in an individual, ineffective or pathological coping mechanisms begin to emerge, with loss of emotional balance, functional capacity, and social adaptation.

Early psychiatrists recognized these problems and their relationship to overwhelming anxiety; thus, anxiety has occupied a central position as an object of study in mental health, especially by the psychoanalytical schools. Early psychoanalytically oriented writings focused on adult neurotic anxiety as a residual of early childhood fears or conflicts. We explained in Chapter 1 that psychoanalytic explanations for adult anxiety reflect Freudian emphasis on difficulties in oral, anal, phallic, oedipal, or genital stages of development. The individual was seen as having partially resolved conflicts at a particular developmental period with resulting incomplete or pathological coping mechanisms, which disguised these long-buried conflicts. Psychoanalysis was the therapeutic process by which the person's thinking and behavior were painstakingly examined to discern long-repressed childhood conflicts, reexamine and reexperience them from an adult perspective, undo pathological coping mechanisms, and develop more adaptive, healthy coping skills.

To a great extent, this internally centered focus on anxiety has been supplanted by the more recent schools of ego psychology and social psychiatry, which view the person as a dynamic, changing individual, interacting with a complex social matrix. The individual is seen as passing psychological milestones in the development of a stable ego structure. These milestones result in the management of normal anxiety in ways which are comfortable for the individual and which promote his or her adaptation to society. Among the best known of these formulations is that of Erik Erikson (1963), which describes eight stages of ego development and their resulting adaptive virtues. According to Erickson, these are:

1. Basic Trust vs. Basic Mistrust: Drive and Hope
2. Autonomy vs. Shame and Doubt: Self Control and Willpower
3. Initiative vs. Guilt: Direction and Purpose
4. Industry vs. Inferiority: Method and Competence
5. Identity vs. Role Confusion: Devotion and Fidelity
6. Intimacy vs. Isolation: Affiliation and Love
7. Generativity vs. Stagnation: Production and Care
8. Ego Integrity vs. Despair: Renunciation and Wisdom

Failure of the individual to complete the work required at the appropriate stage is seen as predisposing her or him to residual ego defects and as diminishing adaptational capacity. For the purpose of the pastoral counselor, the latter formulation seems to offer a more understandable and practical framework. The individual experiences both an internal and an external reality, with spirituality being an active force in both. She or he has an internal being, body, mind, and soul, with the task of finding satisfaction for those components, and she or he has an external societal life encompassing relationships to all other persons and outside forces. Thus, each individual has the complex task of integrating internal and external imperatives even though some of these drives are mutually conflicting. All of these internal and external forces must be kept in a dynamic balance if the ego integrity or functional adaptiveness of the person is to be maintained. However, if internal or external stresses become too great, or if the adaptational capacity of the person is developmentally or constitutionally limited, coping capacity is gradually overwhelmed, and anxiety becomes more and more prominent. It is then that we see the troubled person in need of help with disabling symptoms of anxiety in body, mind, and spirit. Pastoral help may be sought to identify the problem and obtain traditional pastoral care for spiritual strengthening, emotional release and support, sympathetic counseling, and enhancing of adaptational coping skills. The anxious person is a suffering person; yet there is much the pastoral counselor can do as part of the holistic health care team toward the alleviation of anxious suffering and the reestablishment of a healthier physical, emotional, spiritual, and societal equilibrium.

CASE EXAMPLES

Bob

Bob is a thirty-four-year-old graduate student enrolled in a local university. He has sought out pastoral counseling because his wife feels he needs it for a problem related to school. Bob is working on his second doctoral degree and recently announced to his wife his intention to pursue a third in an altogether different area of specialization. His wife has been working for the past thirteen years as a night nurse in a general hospital so Bob could pursue his educational goals and launch a career. They met and married while Bob was in college, and after graduation he began graduate school in history with the goal of becoming a teacher. He was a good student who obtained his MA and subsequently enrolled in a PhD program that took him an additional three years to complete. As the PhD program neared its completion, Bob began having attacks of chest pain and shortness of breath, which necessitated several emergency room visits. No demonstrable organic pathology was found, but Bob was placed on tranquilizers by his local doctor. Because of the frequency of the attacks and the need for medication, Bob felt that he was not ready to function full time as a teacher, so he declined a good job offer with another university and enrolled in a second PhD program in philosophy. His rationale for this was that he could combine history and philosophy into an unusual specialization which would practically guarantee him excellent opportunities with the best universities. Bob applied himself diligently to his new curriculum, and after three years he was nearing completion of his PhD requirements. The chest pains and shortness of breath episodes disappeared for the first two years, but in the final year of his work his symptoms began to reemerge. Again he complained of tight, suffocating chest pain and inability to get his breath. After numerous emergency room visits and physical examinations, Bob and his wife were advised that nothing physical could be found, and that these problems appeared to be psychologically produced stress reactions. One of these occurred on the same day that Bob was to leave for a job interview with a well-known Ivy League college. He felt he had to cancel the interview as a result of his attack. He subsequently advised his wife that he was "not ready" to begin his work as a college teacher, and he stated that he had decided to pursue additional graduate training, this time in political science. As soon as he signed up for this additional training, his symptoms disappeared. Nonetheless, Bob's wife was very dissatisfied with the situation and felt that Bob had a "mental block" which was preventing him from moving ahead with his career goals. She declared herself unwilling to pay for any additional training and insisted that Bob talk to somebody about his problem. Bob himself recognized that his attacks were psychologically based, but he felt that he could not function independently as a teacher until he no longer had symptoms. Thus, he felt obligated to continue his training to avoid further attacks.

Sylvia

Sylvia is a forty-one-year-old woman who has been a lifelong member of your congregation. She was single until two years ago, when she married a previously divorced man who had custody of his three adolescent children. At the time of their marriage, Sylvia was optimistic about taking a maternal role within the family and eager to be a loving mother to these children. Her husband also seemed eager for this to happen, since he was a sales representative for a large manufacturing company and was frequently away from home for long periods of time. The children had had several baby-sitters and relatives supervising them in his absence, but these arrangements seemed temporary at best, and he was eager to provide a more stable home environment for them. Sylvia was attracted to the idea of having an "instant family," and she entered the relationship with high hopes. Strangely, Sylvia, who had always been a consistent participant in church activities, was now seldom in attendance. She seemed isolated and preoccupied, and she no longer volunteered for church duties. One day you happen to see Sylvia in the local grocery store, and in a friendly way you inquire about her health, expressing some concern as to her change in participation. Sylvia replies that she has been unable to participate because of recent severe chronic headaches and backaches that have prevented her from leaving the house as much as in former years. She says she has been receiving various kinds of treatment, including physical therapy, external heat packs, and spinal manipulation, to relieve her discomfort. She says nothing has helped very much, and she hopes you will suggest the name of a reputable doctor. You invite Sylvia to your office for further discussion and make arrangements to see her the following day. The next day at the appointed time Sylvia does not come; instead, a few minutes after the appointed hour, Sylvia calls and explains that once again she cannot leave the home because of a dreadful headache. You note that in the background there seems to be a good deal of commotion, arguing, and yelling. It is apparent that the adolescent children are fighting among themselves, and Sylvia quickly excuses herself with the intention of setting up another appointment at a future time.

Roger

Roger is the fourteen-year-old son of a family in your church. Roger's father is a prominent attorney in your community, and Roger's mother has long been involved in church activities. One day Roger's mother unexpectedly telephones you to say that Roger has recently been involved in a legal problem, and she feels that he needs counseling. You agree to set up an appointment to see Roger and his parents within the next few days. At the appointment, Roger appears nervous, sullen, and withdrawn. His parents are clearly angry with him, and they readily describe the nature of their concerns. Roger has recently been arrested for shoplifting in a local stereo equipment store. He was caught with a small compact disc player in his jacket. Roger's father admits that this was not the first time Roger had been caught shoplifting, but that for the past year or two there had been several incidents of Roger's stealing small items from stereo and record stores. Because of Roger's father's status in the community, he has been able to "fix" many of these earlier charges and settle things out of court with no publicity or criminal record for Roger. The most recently involved storeowner, however, said that he intended to press charges and was not going to let the matter drop. Roger's parents are furious over the embarrassment this has brought, and they are also concerned because their repeated warnings to Roger about these consequences have gone unheeded. His parents also say that Roger does not have any stolen merchandise at home. In fact, they are altogether unclear as to what he does with it after he steals it. When caught, he reports that he intends to give the merchandise away to his friends, and some parental detective work showed that this was indeed the case. He had given away many items to classmates and neighborhood friends. No trades, money exchanges, or drugs appeared to be involved in these "gift" transactions. Because of obvious parental anger, the parents are asked to leave the room for a brief time to allow for a private discussion with Roger. He says he does not know why he steals these things, but notes he has been doing this more and more in the past two years. He feels at times overcome by an "irresistible urge," and then he steals an item and gives it to a friend. Roger usually retires to the friend's house where he listens to the radio, or the two of them may share the equipment for many hours over the next several weeks. When asked how he can conceal these activities and the time spent on them from his parents, Roger says that his parents have been preoccupied with problems of their own. Initially vague and defensive, Roger eventually begins to cry and says that, in spite of its stable outward appearance, his family is in great turmoil with parental divorce imminent. He cannot be sure exactly what is happening, but it appears his father has taken up a relationship with another woman, probably his secretary, and that he has been spending more and more time away from home. When the parents are together at home, constant accusations and much conflict occur. If he is around the house while this is going on, he retires to his room and frequently becomes ill, sometimes even vomiting from anxiety. His way of coping is to get out of the house and spend as much time as he can in the homes of friends. He has learned that gifts, even if they are stolen, will usually ensure acceptance and allow him to stay at a friend's house as long as possible. Roger admits that his grades have declined in school and that he has been cutting classes lately because he dreads the embarrassment of being behind in his studies.

Celia

Celia is a thirty-five-year-old woman referred to you by a local psychiatrist for pastoral counseling. The psychiatrist advises you that Celia has been involved in a marriage which has proven to be very traumatic, and that she feels hopeless and trapped. She has had innumerable psychosomatic medical problems and frequently sees medical doctors in emergency rooms for various aches and pains, menstrual difficulties, insomnia, and other symptoms. At the time of Celia's visit with you, she is nervous and hyperactive. She paces around the study, saying she needs a cigarette. She begins the session by complaining that she cannot find a doctor who will pay attention to her serious medical problems, and she says that her psychiatrist has recommended a divorce. This is contrary to her religious beliefs, and she is fearful of the unknown and of financial independence. She says that the psychiatrist and many of her family members feel she is suffering because of her husband. She claims that her husband is a compulsive gambler who is constantly preoccupied with placing bets on various sporting events. He has numerous bookies whom he constantly telephones, and he is secretive about financial matters at home. She complains of constant worry and anxiety from his gambling compulsion. She knows when her husband has made a big bet because he is irritable, argumentative, and preoccupied. His personality changes, which are dramatic, have been going on for many years. She feels that she and her children have suffered because of his compulsion. On occasion, money has had to be diverted from family essentials to pay off gambling debts. Her husband has borrowed money from friends and relatives to make ends meet during these times, and recently he forged her name on several bank loan agreements to obtain money. All of this is making her a "nervous wreck," but she feels paralyzed by her religious upbringing, by her children's need to have a father present, and by her own lack of self-confidence. She has worked with two psychiatrists in the past, neither of whom could involve her husband in therapy. Both they and all of her family members and friends have repeatedly recommended that she divorce her husband, but she has not been able to bring herself to do this.

RECOGNITION

Anxiety per se is not necessarily a pathological emotion. Moderate levels of anxiety are commonly experienced by everyone in the course of normal day-to-day existence. Anxiety serves a useful function as a warning or a sentinel emotion, protecting us from uncomfortable, distressing, or even dangerous circumstances. Low levels of anxiety add to the excitement, challenge, and exhilaration of daily living. Attempts to avoid even normal levels of anxiety may lead to character regression and self-absorption, psychosis (flight into non-reality), chronic narcosis with drugs or alcohol, or social isolation.

When normal levels of anxiety are exceeded by conflict-producing internal or external demands, anxious suffering or pathological anxiety becomes evident. The anxiety becomes disabling if it is extremely frequent or constant; if it produces pathological changes in the person's body, mind, soul, or social interactions; if coping skills are overwhelmed; if healthy defenses are replaced by ineffective or inappropriate ones; or if the anxiety is far out of proportion to the apparent stimulus. Manifestations of severe anxiety are highly individualized. Symptoms of anxiety vary widely depending on physical, emotional, spiritual, and behavioral factors within each individual.

People who are aware of their anxiety complain that they feel worried, nervous, or tense. They may or may not be able to identify the internal or external causes of stress. In general, these individuals are more "psychologically minded" than most people and can usually, with reflective counseling and consistent encouragement, analyze their own problems, mobilize their coping skills, and work through their anxieties. More challenging circumstances arise, however, when anxious people have little awareness of the psychological nature of their suffering. They may not be at all aware that they are nervous, worried, or tense, and, in fact, externally may not appear to be so. Generally, such individuals have more subtle indicators of anxiety, in the form of physical manifestations and behavior change. Physical changes, which can be barely detectable without medical examination, may include muscle tension and perhaps spasm in neck, back, legs, and even in the involuntary musculature, such as bowel or vocal cord muscles. Functional disturbance may range from mild muscle fatigue with physical aches and pains to spasm and structural breakdown. Band-type headaches and spasm-related backaches are common. Internally, indigestion, excess stomach acid, spastic cramping, and diarrhea are often seen. These gastrointestinal symptoms may worsen to include ulcers, tissue erosion, and bleeding, which require medical or surgical intervention.

Anxious patients usually show marked evidence of generalized central nervous system overstimulation. In addition to their tense appearance, they may appear irritable and short-tempered or hurried or pressured in their speech, often with a quavering voice or stammering. Nervous fidgeting or pacing is often seen. Difficulty sleeping may be reported, as well as frequent nightmares and fear dreams (often with symbolization and condensation of unconsciously feared stimuli). So-called hyperventilation symptoms are frequent. These may include a feeling of vertigo, shortness of breath, inability to catch the breath or get enough air, a sense of smothering, tightening of the throat or chest, lump in the throat, or numbness of the fingers or mouth. Rapid pulse rates, elevations of blood pressure, excessive perspiration, and hand tremor are also common. Since many of these symptoms accompany physical illnesses such as heart attacks, a thorough evaluation by a physician is indicated when physical symptoms are present.

ASSESSMENT OF SEVERITY

The severity of anxious suffering is roughly proportional to the degree of functional impairment. Most people with moderate levels of anxiety can function in normal routines with barely noticeable impairment. As anxious suffering worsens, however, subjective complaints of tension, worry, dread, or anxiety are seen. The person in distress may repeatedly call the pastor, physician, psychiatrist, or hospital emergency room. The frequency and emotional intensity of the calls may well indicate the person's degree of subjective discomfort and need for help. Typically, insomnia, muscle aches and pains, and other physical symptoms are very distressing. Fears and apprehensions are exaggerated, and usual coping mechanisms fail. Marked severity of anxious suffering is indicated if the patient's usual coping mechanisms, including prayer, are ineffective or unavailable to him or her, or if there are self-defeating attempts to obtain relief or escape through violence, suicide, running away, vandalism, shoplifting, or other behavioral channels. Anxiety may be considered severe if there is recent, inappropriate self-medication with alcohol and drugs, which may reflect exhaustion of the person's own internal coping strength. Greater severity is also indicated by a history of previous psychiatric treatment or psychiatric hospitalization.

CRISIS INTERVENTION

People suffering from anxiety are usually looking for strength, stability, and sympathy for their distress. The pastoral counselor should react to the crisis with unflustered calm, poise, caring, concern, and understanding. Place the anxious person in a calm, quiet environment, such as the pastor's study or office, and allow no interruptions while dealing with him or her. Be sympathetic about the person's suffering and discomfort; these are genuine and distressing even if the fears are exaggerated.

The person should be encouraged to "talk it out" with the pastor in an open, honest discussion of all the issues. This discussion is usually best accomplished by a brief, chronological review of the person's life history or, if this is well known to the minister, at least a review of all the facts surrounding the present crisis. This review should exclude nothing. It should cover all relevant details—past, present, and future—that determine or reveal the person's exposure to stresses and his or her pattern of coping with them. Because of the natural human difficulty in self-evaluation, the opinions of the person's significant others, such as spouse, employers, and parents, should be requested. If adequate pains have been taken to get this background information, usually a rational plan can be formulated to obtain help. The importance of this historical data cannot be overstated. It is extremely difficult to recognize anxiety, assess its severity, and formulate a helping plan without adequate background information.

The process of talking it out and sharing this background information can have a remarkable cathartic effect. The pastoral counselor is quietly building a helping alliance with the suffering person and nonverbally communicating a message of understanding, concern, and willingness to help. This helping alliance is vitally important to the recovery process and ideally should include all members of the holistic health care team. The suffering person receives a message of hope: "Help is available for you." Restoration of physical, emotional, spiritual, and social equilibrium can be accomplished by mobilizing whatever resources are necessary within the health care team.

Background information may reveal that the patient's reported anxiety is only a camouflage emotion for other distressing, but embarrassing, emotions such as rage, anger, aggression, jealousy, or depression. A careful review of the individual's history will usually bring these hidden emotions to light. The cause of the anxious distress may be readily apparent, or it may be well hidden, necessitating more prolonged, intensive exploration by a mental health professional. The adaptive capacity of the individual is usually clarified by the historical review. Typical coping mechanisms, strengths, and weaknesses are identified and provide the structure for the therapeutic plan of enhancing strengths and avoiding weaknesses. One of the distressing aspects of dealing with anxious persons is their normal human tendency to complain bitterly but at the same time to resist change and fail to follow advice. Thus, honesty and openness on the patient's part are not sufficient for long-term relief of symptoms. Willingness is an essential component of a healthy attitude; the person must be willing to listen, to change her or his thinking and behavior, and to accept help in whatever form offered.

Psychiatric referral and possible hospitalization are indicated for signs of extreme or unrelenting anxiety. Such signs may include marked functional impairment with deterioration of occupational or personal responsibilities; behavioral symptoms such as running away, vandalism, and petty theft; self-destructive behavior; suicidal thinking; or reality breaks. If outpatient or ambulatory counseling has not improved the patient's symptoms after a few weeks and if stress remains high, professional referral is probably indicated. Hospitalization may serve many purposes for the anxious person. He or she will usually obtain a comprehensive physical evaluation with laboratory studies, which will physically demonstrate anxiety-related changes, such as nervous system arousal. In addition, the examination will usually allay fears about the presence of more serious disease or impending death. In addition, hospitalization allows isolation from the overwhelming demands of the environment or stress-producing situation. This isolation may grant patients some temporary rest from the conflict, while allowing them to reconstitute and mobilize their defenses with the support of the entire holistic health care team.

Medications, especially tranquilizers and sedatives, are not always indicated but may help if the anxiety is severe, if there is functional impairment, or if there is loss of contact with reality. Most physicians are aware of the danger of addiction from long-term use of "minor" tranquilizers and sedatives and thus tend to use them for brief periods of time at lower dosage levels. Medication management is always a medical decision, but this does not preclude strengthening the anxious person's internal resources for coping with reality. Such is the role of the supportive psychotherapies and/or of pastoral counseling. When the person is more stable and in better control of his or her emotions, the need for medication may be less pressing, but the goal of the pastoral counselor should be the person's utilization of all the health resources at his or her disposal.

While the anxious patient is in the hospital, the helping alliance with the pastoral counselor should be maintained. Anxious people need patient, frequent reassurance and explanations, even if these seem repetitive. Any sign that shows the patient your interest, concern, and involvement is for the good. These signs of interest may include taking her or him to the hospital, being there at the time of admission, visiting, phoning, or giving pamphlets, a bible, or other reading materials. Use your helping alliance to facilitate the patient's care: "Let's tell the doctor about your fear of . . ." Facing the feared reality alone is often the paralyzing apprehension of anxious people. Reassurance that you, the spiritual community, the medical team, and God are available to help is very powerful.

People in acute anxious stress may be irritable or angry because of their suffering and because of the failure of others around them, including the health care team, to relieve their suffering when and how they would like it done. The pastoral counselor is advised to avoid taking sides in conflict situations or legitimizing unreasonable demands or inappropriate behaviors.

Prayer for the anxious person can take many forms. The minister can assist him or her in prayer, and therein develop trust in a loving and beneficent God. Prayers for hope, as well as for serene acceptance of God's will and wisdom, are timely. Prayers for internal peace, calm, serenity, strength, and the courage and willingness to cooperate are recommended. Recognition of God's protection and love is an additional useful theme.

The anxious person can use other therapeutic modalities that offer variety but may also come with a confusing degree of freedom in obtaining help. Psychoanalysis, that is, long-term, in-depth, uncovering psychotherapy, has the advantage of generally assuring the patient a reputable therapist, since analytical training is very rigorous and well supervised. Its disadvantages are high cost, frequent sessions, and theoretical bias.

Hypnosis may be administered by hypnotists with variable degrees of training and experience. It is not considered a medical treatment unless administered by a medical or mental health care professional. It may offer some relief from milder forms of anxiety, but often such improvements are short-lived. Reputable medical professional organizations should be consulted if one is seeking a therapist who specializes in hypnosis.

Biofeedback is a useful technological tool for the diagnosis and management of anxiety-related symptoms. Instruments measure levels of nervous system tension, and then the machine feeds this information back to patients so they are able to perceive their level of stress and consciously reduce it. Biofeedback would seem to be particularly applicable to anxiety states manifested by muscular tension, such as frequent headaches or backache. Other applications are possible for panic attacks and phobias of all kinds.

Group therapy is a psychotherapeutic modality in which a number of people meet together to deal with emotional and behavioral problems. Some advantages of this technique are lower cost, greater opportunity to work on interpersonal skills, peer guidance, support, and confrontation. Some disadvantages include diminished contact with the primary therapist, difficulties in getting the right mix of people, and greater confrontation than in individual therapy.

Last, phobia clinics are currently receiving a great deal of publicity for management of anxiety symptoms. All "new" developments in mental health should be regarded with a degree of skepticism; yet, these clinics do seem to provide benefit for certain people. Their best outcomes seem to relate to well-defined fear situations, such as fears of airplanes, escalators, elevators, leaving home, or driving a car. These isolated fears may or may not have unconscious neurotic determinants and are usually amenable to straightforward behavioral modification and gradual desensitization techniques. These clinics excel at providing such techniques and offer the phobic person an opportunity to confront the feared situation gradually with the support of an experienced worker. Disadvantages are related to the lack of professionalism of many phobia clinics, as well as to the limited training and experience of their personnel. Also, phobia clinics do not seem appropriate for more severe, generalized anxiety problems, or for those with complicated psychodynamic or situational determinants.

Physical exercise is probably one of the most underrated modalities for anxiety reduction. It has the advantage of being a physiologic treatment; that is, it does not involve artificial agents or even aggressive psychological treatment. It converts internally felt muscle tension into the satisfying outlet of motor activity. The resulting fatigue is natural and sleep-inducing. Studies have demonstrated that physical exercise is effective in reducing anxiety and tension.

COUNSELING IN THE RECOVERY PHASE

Counseling of the anxious person in the postcrisis phase is primarily directed at maintenance of functioning, with secondary attention to moderation of anxiety. All counseling efforts should be directed at returning the person to active functioning as soon as possible and to maintaining that functioning, consistent with the patient's realistic capabilities, in spite of anxious discomfort. Usually, anxious patients have a tendency to let their anxious symptoms and fears control and immobilize them. Typically, they will feel they cannot return to work, home, or other routine responsibilities *until they feel better.* They will come to you and their doctors with the challenge to help them feel better so they can return to normal activity, yet there is an obvious difficulty in this request. They are asking you to help with emotional discomfort over which neither they nor you have any apparent control. Since little control over emotion is possible, residual anxiety leads to paralysis of will and impaired functioning. This paralysis leads to further functional regression and avoidance of anxiety-producing situations, such as job or school. An additional problem is fear of the return of the anxiety, that is, fear and anticipation of this discomfort even before it is felt. When this attitude becomes a chronic one, the anxious person becomes a neurotic whose rehabilitation to full functioning is difficult. Healthy action must precede healthy thinking. Anxious people must "act their way into good thinking."

The appropriate way to circumvent this cycle in the recovery phase is through taking the behavior-oriented approach by placing primary emphasis on becoming active, and by returning to full responsibility regardless of whether one feels that anxiety will permit it. When the impairment is mild, this return to full functioning can proceed very quickly, for example, in returning to work immediately after hospitalization. On the other hand, with chronicity and long-term anxiety-produced maladjustment, a gradual phasing in of responsibilities may be needed. Fear is overcome by gradual, persistent familiarity with the feared object or situation. The person must take initiative in confronting the situation at some level, even in the most modest degree, and must continually repeat that exposure until it becomes comfortable. When that exposure is easily managed, additional exposure and more responsibility can be sought. The counselor should always resist the patient's tendency to avoid anxiety-provoking situations, unless their management is beyond the patient's ability or avoiding them involves no functional impairment. Instead, the counselor should take an encouraging, facilitating, and strengthening position with the person. This behavioral approach with an emphasis on action first and relief of anxiety later is summarized in many therapeutic slogans that are widely used by mental health practitioners. Among these are "Function through it," "Act your way into good thinking," and "Move the muscles."

Improvement in chronic anxious suffering is seldom achieved in a short time. Most anxious people have suffered with their symptoms for years, and recovery with emotional strengthening is usually a long-term process. Emphasis is always on gradual character building and strengthening by persistent, gradual acceptance of responsibility with the help of others. The anxious person usually needs the support of others to persevere in his or her recovery plan. The support of family members, church, clergypeople, mental health professionals, self-help groups, employers, friends, and others is valuable. Recovery, Inc., and Emotions Anonymous are the two self-help groups that are often helpful for anxious persons. The book *Mental Health Through Will-Training* by Dr. Abraham A. Low (1977) is used by members of Recovery, Inc., and is available in local bookstores. The clerical counselor can act as a catalyst to mobilize supportive social networks around anxious sufferers to keep them on a path of gradual improvement, in spite of their tendency toward avoidance and regression.

Chronic worriers can be helped to face life "one day at a time" or even "one hour at a time" to mobilize all their coping resources for a finite period, rather than for the indefinite future. These short units of time soon add up, and the anxious person can then reflect on the satisfaction of having "made it" for weeks, months, or years. The resulting optimism becomes a self-fulfilling prophecy that perpetuates re-covery.

The normal human tendency to regress and relapse into old ways of thinking and acting is always present. Pathological devices for anxiety reduction are always a temptation for the anxious person. Fleeing and avoidance are common, as are other escapes from ten-sion, such as drugs, alcohol, or suicide. Running from responsibility-oriented therapy almost ensures continuation of the illness and is therefore self-destructive. The pastoral counselor should watch for early tendencies toward regression and repetition of old styles of thinking and behavior, alert the patient, and encourage him or her toward healthier coping.

Prayer, scriptural reading, and spiritual guidance are indispensable components of such pastoral counseling. Prayer can focus on a search for serenity with its acceptance of things beyond our control. Free-dom from worry, dread, and fear can be alleviated through conscious contact with God and a newly developing faith and trust in His watch-ful beneficence.

Chapter 4

The Chemically Dependent Person

OVERVIEW

Chemical dependency, meaning alcoholism, drug addiction, or both, is an extremely common illness today. We are experiencing a worldwide epidemic of chemical dependencies, and the most likely cause is pervasive acceptance of these substances into every aspect of our lives. Drinking alcohol is such a commonplace activity now that it can be said to be the lubricant of most social activity in the United States. In addition, the ready availability of mood-altering substances, uppers, downers, and painkillers has put temporary, chemically assisted mood and behavior change within the reach of everyone. Regrettably, it appears that technologically we have outrun our moral and philosophical guidelines regarding the use of these powerful substances. Appropriate therapeutic use, much less recreational use, is not easily defined. With the proliferation of these substances in our daily lives, casualties are almost inevitable. In 1991, the National Household Survey on Drug Abuse found that 12.8 percent of Americans, or 26 million, had tried an illegal drug during that year (Office of Applied Studies at SAMHSA, 1999). As of 1998, the percentages of Americans who had used drugs or binged on alcohol during the previous month were as follows: marijuana 5 percent, cocaine 0.8 percent, crack 0.2 percent, heroin 0.1 percent, and alcohol (binge) 15.6 percent. Factors relating to substance abuse are now the fourth leading cause of death in the United States. Over one million people received treatment for substance abuse in 1998 (U.S. Bureau of the Census, 2000). Current estimates of the economic devastation caused by alcoholism and drug abuse are in excess of $80 billion per year for the United States. Alcohol or substance abuse is now the number one cause of death (including homicide) for people under thirty. Approximately 60 percent of violent crime in this country is related to alcohol and/or drugs. Nearly everyone knows someone whose life has been profoundly affected, directly or indirectly, by substance abuse or dependency.

The United States is now experiencing a dramatic change in its problems with alcohol. Alcoholism used to be thought of as an older person's disease. In years past it was rare to find anyone under the age of forty-five at an Alcoholics Anonymous meeting. Now almost half of the people who come to AA for the first time are under twenty-five, and many are in their teens. Formerly, alcoholism was thought of as a man's disease; now approximately half of the new alcoholics who enter treatment are women.

In addition, the widespread availability of mood-altering substances has expanded our understanding of alcoholism, which should now more correctly be called chemical dependency, since drugs are frequently a coexistent problem. The following cases serve to highlight certain aspects of chemical dependency.

CASE EXAMPLES

Richard

Richard is a forty-four-year-old manufacturer's representative for a local company. He is responsible for sales in a broad geographic area and spends much of his time traveling. His business involves a good deal of client entertainment and socializing. He and his wife come to see you because of marital problems. She reports that in the past six months he has become moody, irritable, and argumentative. Whereas formerly Richard was very even tempered, now relatively small things trigger outbursts of rage. On one occasion, he directed his temper toward his wife and pushed her down the stairs, breaking her arm. They both went to the local emergency room and, in order to conceal what had really happened, made up a story about an accidental fall. Richard claims that the next day he had no recollection of what had occurred. He acknowledges that during these episodes he had been drinking "a few beers," but denies vehemently that he was drunk. His wife states that Richard's changes of personality always occur while he is drinking, and that when he is not drinking, he is a very pleasant fellow. Richard denies that drinking has been a serious problem; rather, he feels that he has been under considerable psychological stress lately since business has not been as good as it used to be. He claims that the company is pressuring him. Asked about his past performance at work, he says that he has always been an excellent performer, and was in the past regarded as having executive potential. He feels that the company has recently betrayed him because he was passed over for a promotion, and another person was advanced ahead of him. He claims to be depressed from these events and feels that indeed he has been drinking more than before, but that this should pass when his depression about these events lifts.

Richard's changes of mood and personality have had a very negative effect on his marriage, and his wife is now thinking of separation, even divorce.

Kelly

Kelly, the fifty-six-year-old wife of a local corporate executive, was for years a prominent and active member of your congregation. Nonetheless, for the past year or so, she has dropped out of sight. Inquiries to her friends and associates indicate that she has not been feeling well and has been under a doctor's care. Deciding to pay her a pastoral call of assistance, you go to her home. Although it is 3:00 in the afternoon, Kelly comes to the door in her pajamas. Her speech is slurred and her grooming is poor, far out of character for her normal personality. She informs you that she has not been well, and that she has been under a doctor's care for "nervous spells." When you inquire as to the identity of the doctor she is seeing, she becomes evasive. Concerned about her appearance and change of personality, you invite her and her husband to your office. In the office three days later, Kelly looks dramatically different. She is neat and well groomed, and attempts to convey an impression of health and contentment. Her husband is not quite so sanguine. He says that about a year ago, Kelly began having bizarre seizurelike episodes which necessitated several hospitalizations. Some of these hospitalizations were medical, and some were psychiatric. During these spells, Kelly appeared to go into a convulsion. Nothing could be found on medical workup, but according to her husband, one of her early physicians believed that her spells were a type of withdrawal reaction, possibly from alcohol or medication. When he suggested treatment for chemical dependency in a specialized rehabilitation center, Kelly would have nothing further to do with him. Her husband fears she has some kind of emotional problem that she is attempting to deal with through high doses of medication. He fears that she has been seeing several doctors at once. She typically sees a doctor and impresses him with her emotional distress, coming away with prescriptions for mood-altering medications. By seeing several doctors at once, she has been able to maintain a more or less constant supply of potent medicines. When a doctor begins to catch on to what she is doing, she drops him or her and goes to another. Most recently, her husband does not even know how many doctors are involved, but he has been finding empty medication bottles throughout the house. They are in her shoes, in her clothing, in the bedsheets, in the kitchen, everywhere. He cannot recall when he last observed her in an unmedicated or fully alert state. Her spells or convulsions generally occur when she goes out in public for a while, and he believes that she stops her medication prior to going out. He thinks it is entirely possible she had withdrawal reactions during those times. When asked if he feels his wife is medication dependent or addicted, he replies, "A year ago I didn't think so, but I can see it now." He is afraid that unless she gets off of the pills she will lose her marriage and perhaps even her life.

Lisa

Lisa is a nineteen-year-old sophomore at a local college. She is the daughter of a family that has been in your church for many years. Although Lisa was formerly a model student, her parents now report she is experiencing serious difficulty and has been sent home by her college. Lisa was an all-around good girl until about two and one-half years ago in high school, when she began associating with some students who took drugs. Her behavior and attitude changed dramatically after that, and she began getting involved in petty difficulties at the end of her senior year. She missed class frequently, and on two occasions she was sent home because she was "ill." Her mother suspects these illnesses were the result of intoxication. Lately Lisa's grades in college have been dismal. The college informed her parents that Lisa has seldom been in class and has fallen far behind her classmates. She was finally sent home when she was picked up on campus wandering around stuporously in a state of partial undress at 4:00 a.m. She had no idea where she was, and she had to be hospitalized for observation. Doctors reported that blood tests revealed numerous medications and street drugs. Lisa sits quietly during the interview up until this time, and then begins to answer questions. She does not deny using drugs, including marijuana, cocaine, sedatives, alcohol, and diet pills, but she feels completely justified in doing so since she believes that this is an entirely normal thing to do, and that all of her friends are doing it. She can see no difference between use of these medications and social drinking for her parents. Her parents report that they have seen some of Lisa's school associates, and that most of them are "troublemakers" who are having serious problems with school and the law. Her parents are concerned about where Lisa obtains money to purchase drugs, and as a protective measure they have kept her on a very meager allowance. The parents subsequently learn from a friend that one of Lisa's boyfriends has been selling drugs, and that on occasion Lisa helps him do so.

RECOGNITION

Recognition of the problem of chemical dependency may or may not be an easy matter, since very often the problem is disguised as something else. The patient may wish to conceal the problem out of fear, shame, or embarrassment, or in order to continue access to the pleasure-giving substances. Denial of the extent of the problem is commonplace. Another problem in recognition is the matter of defining chemical dependency. Alcoholism, chemical dependency, drug abuse, and addiction are difficult to recognize and quantify. Although some people believe *any* recreational substance use is a problem, more stringent criteria for chemical dependency are needed to separate the "social" or recreational users who are not harmfully involved from those who are victimized by use of these substances.

In order to clarify definition and facilitate recognition, it may be helpful to use alcoholism as the model of a chemical dependency problem. What is alcoholism anyway? How do we know if someone is alcoholic or not? Is it possible to be an alcoholic if one drinks only on weekends or if drinking does not interfere with one's work? What about people who claim they can quit whenever they want to?

It is useful at this juncture to ascertain how professionals in the field of chemical dependency make this diagnosis. The crux of the matter is that they feel alcohol is an addictive drug, and alcoholism is addiction to it. Chemical dependencies, by extension, are similarly diseases of addiction. Although alcoholics can be from any walk of life, educational level, or social status, once the disease begins to manifest itself, a predictable pattern of behavior and thinking will begin to emerge. The diagnosis is based on the presence or absence of these alcoholic patterns of thinking and behavior. The difficulty in diagnosis is that alcoholism is characterized by loss of control over a substance. Loss of control is never easy to observe or measure. We have no psychological tests for loss of control, and chemical laboratory studies may or may not help. Since the affected person often does not wish to acknowledge loss of control or may not even see it, how are we able to discern it? We recognize alcoholism (and other chemical dependencies) through observation of the *consequences* of loss of control, that is, by perceiving alcoholic thinking, behavior, and other consequences of the disease. In fact, we are forced to rely on the assumption that "Where there's smoke, there's fire," and thus deduce that when the consequences of out-of-control drinking are repeatedly present, loss of control is indeed the problem.

What are the diagnostic patterns of alcoholic thinking and behavior, and what are the telltale consequences of loss of control? For most people, there is an initial period of nonproblematic drinking. Indeed, the person begins to appreciate the wonderful efficacy of the drug. He or she experiences tranquilization, relaxation, or euphoria, and begins to feel that he or she is more outgoing, talkative, amusing, socially interesting, or sexually appealing. Negative occurrences are forgotten through euphoric recall. Alcohol may be used to induce relaxation or sleep. In short, it is an excellent drug, and the person soon learns to benefit from it. Gradually, however, the phenomenon of tolerance begins to show itself; the individual must keep raising the dose in order to achieve the desired effect. Eventually the beneficial dose becomes the intoxicating dose as well. Simultaneous with this development of physical tolerance people experience an alteration in their thinking about it, so there is a psychological component to their increased use. They begin to feel that if a little alcohol helps somewhat, then a bit more will work even better. Also, they begin to feel not only that they are functioning better under the influence, but also that they cannot function nearly so well without it. Indeed, they begin to rely on alcohol even in anticipation of stressful circumstances or social events. For example, the housewife who begins by having a drink to fortify herself for her daily chores and activities may soon begin to feel that she cannot function at all without a drink. Eventually, she comes to feel that she cannot do her chores and activities at all whether she has a drink or not, and the alcohol then merely provides a chemical escape from her intolerable burdens.

Slowly and insidiously, the person's pattern of drinking begins to change. From periodic, nonharmful social drinking or relief drinking, there is more and more frequent reliance on alcohol for the effect or for mood alteration. The person comes to enjoy the effects of alcohol and wants it more and more often. Since this much drinking is generally frowned upon by others, the person begins to take some pains to conceal the amount or the consequences of the drinking. All sorts of surreptitious means to maintain access to alcohol may be employed. Bottles that are stored in the home for guests may be drunk from and then reconstituted with water to make them appear as though no liquor is missing. Bottles may be hidden around the house to provide access when no one is looking, and empties (always a problem to remove discreetly) may be hidden as well. Any kind of cover-up or dishonesty about the amount, frequency, or consequences of drinking is virtually diagnostic of a serious problem.

Generally, once this increase has occurred, the first negative consequences are in the areas of marriage and job. The person often becomes inattentive to normal responsibilities, and household duties or employment-related tasks are neglected. There may be profound personality changes, frequently described as "Dr. Jekyll and Mr. Hyde" alterations. When sober, the person may be relaxed, kind, cheerful, and pleasant. When drinking, a profound alteration may occur, resulting in nastiness, irritability, and even potential violence to self or others. The spouse may become progressively more intolerant of the excessive drinking and mood changes, and more distrustful of the drinker's credibility, as the lies and deceptions begin to mount. The drinker becomes progressively more irresponsible about domestic matters, with the result that the spouse must carry more and more responsibility. With the abdication of responsibility comes a loss of authority, and soon neither the children nor the spouse is paying any attention to the alcoholic's attempts to exert authority in the home. The resulting frustration may increase the drinker's violent displays of temper.

Typically, the nonalcoholic spouse becomes more resentful, angry, and fearful, and she or he may try threats or bribery to get the alcoholic to modify her or his behavior. Such maneuvers are only temporarily successful. The alcoholic goes "on the wagon" for a short period of time but soon begins to feel that he or she can handle "one or two," and the drinking compulsion is triggered anew. Episodes of intoxication become more and more frequent, and often alcoholic blackouts occur. These are alcohol-induced memory lapses that happen after a period of heavy drinking. In a typical example, the alcoholic will be drinking heavily in the evening, and then black out on the following day and forget all the events of that drinking period. He or she may have called distant relatives late at night while under the influence ("telephonitis"). Or his or her behavior may have been violent and nasty. He or she may have wrecked or lost the car on the way home. Such occurrences become more frequent, and the alcoholic may begin to believe that he or she is going insane.

The alcoholic begins experiencing considerable social pressure to cut down or control it. This pressure may come from spouse, parents, children, close friends, physician, or employer. What they all fail to realize is that the person has gone beyond the point where control is possible. In other words, the individual does well as long as he or she is totally abstinent from alcohol and similar substances. Reintroducing any of these chemicals into the system restimulates his or her addiction trigger, and a slip begins that usually progresses rapidly back to his or her old pattern of excessive, out-of-control intake. After he or she makes several attempts at control, everyone is disgusted with the alcoholic, and the alcoholic is disgusted with himself or herself. Nonetheless, he or she can scarcely conceive of quitting altogether. The individual's life is now centered on alcohol. He or she has abandoned hobbies, sports, and normal family pastimes and activities, and concentrates his or her efforts around satisfaction of the desire for continued drinking.

The alcoholic's associates are now almost exclusively heavy drinkers. He or she is embarrassed to be around nondrinking friends. In fact, they are quite embarrassed to be around the alcoholic, since they do not know exactly what to say. They may feel helpless and frustrated in watching the changes that occur right before their eyes.

Usually, there is a concerted attempt to protect the job from the effects of drinking. Nonetheless, the effects of chronic, heavy use eventually begin to affect job performance, and often absenteeism, with numerous minor medical excuses, is the chief manifestation. Frequently, the spouse is asked to call in sick for the alcoholic, usually when the person is still intoxicated, hungover, or drinking. After a while, the spouse tires of lying and covering up, so the alcoholic makes the calls. Eventually, the alcoholic does not bother calling anymore. Output falls dramatically, and warnings and eventual dismissal usually result.

Experience has shown that the best motivation for the alcoholic to seek help is coercive pressure, with threat of job loss, from the employer. Often, probationary strategies contingent upon long-term involvement in a rigorous treatment program will successfully motivate the alcoholic. However, such employer pressure is not always available. Sometimes the alcoholic has already lost his or her job and is unemployed, or the person may be an executive accountable to no one or have no outside employer, as with students or housewives. Absence of such a coercive factor is a definite hindrance to motivation, and this places more pressure on family members to supply the tough love and motivation for seeking treatment. Many large companies have employee assistance programs that help employees and family members obtain professional, competent help for a variety of problems, including alcoholism and chemical dependency. Many employers have an enlightened attitude about drinking problems and are not eager to get rid of problem drinkers in the workforce. In fact, many problem drinkers are valued employees, and generally the company simply wants the person sober, rehabilitated, and back to work.

In the meantime, our alcoholic is progressing still further with the disease and manifesting additional problems. Because of frequent mood changes, depression, and irritability, psychiatric help or counseling may be sought. Often the extent of drinking is concealed from the doctor, and if the doctor does become aware of it and attempts to motivate the person, the reaction may be to find a new doctor. Legal problems may begin as the person accumulates charges of drunk driving and alcohol-related automotive accidents. Such charges create additional financial hardship on an already-strained alcoholic home, since the alcoholic must now pay for high-risk category auto insurance, attorney fees, hospitalizations, lawsuits, and replacement of automobiles.

Financial problems are a consistent feature of an alcoholic home because of unemployment, mounting bills, and general neglect of personal financial responsibility. Continued purchase of alcohol and drugs also creates a heavy and continuous drain on family finances. Eventually the family may be forced to protect the money supply by picking up paychecks, doling out modest allowances, and confiscating credit cards. Wages may be garnished and financial stress may be extreme.

More common still is overall neglect of all responsibility and general collapse of the person's life and that of those around her or him. It is estimated that the alcoholic seriously affects four or more persons, particularly her or his family. Typical family responses include embarrassed avoidance of friends and outside associates or, conversely, going home may be so painful that there is extensive involvement in all sorts of outside activities. Friends are seldom invited in to visit, since the behavior of the alcoholic may be unpredictable or obnoxious.

Attempts to control drinking may include addiction substitutes, such as tranquilizers or sedatives. These may be supplied by well-intentioned doctors who feel that these medications are at least better than alcohol. Unfortunately, however, the addictive compulsion forces the chemically dependent person to increase the dose or drink alcohol with the medications, or to employ several doctors simultaneously. Alcoholics and addictive mood-altering medications do not mix.

Spiritual problems may be profound. Marked personality changes with moral and spiritual deterioration may occur. The person becomes apathetic or hostile toward church and previously valued spiritual activities, and his or her alcohol-related conduct may be immoral. Gambling, infidelity, and violence are common. The person may suffer from profound embarrassment, stigma, and self-loathing. Guilt may be acute. Withdrawal from the spiritual community usually results because continued scrutiny from friends and associates is so painful. The person may feel completely lost, hopeless, and abandoned even by God. Hatred of God under these circumstances is not uncommon. Suicide, frequently contemplated, is often a danger and is one of the most common causes of death of alcoholics and chemical dependents.

Physical collapse may ensue with an amazing array of alcohol-induced medical conditions. Alcoholism may be the significant precipitating factor in cirrhosis, pancreatitis, gastritis, ulcers, hypertension, tuberculosis, cancer, seizures, psychiatric illness, and trauma of every conceivable kind. Alcohol-related disease, disability, or injury accounts for a sizeable percentage of the daily census of virtually every hospital in the United States. Yet in spite of frequent medical warnings, the untreated person will continue to drink and deteriorate. Early death through accident or illness is the rule rather than the exception. The average life expectancy for unrecovered alcoholics is approximately fifty-six years. The average age of death due to cirrhosis of the liver is thirty-nine. Professionals in the field of alcoholism recognize the illness as a potentially fatal, self-perpetuating, yet treatable disease. Alcoholism is a serious, life-threatening illness in which the pastoral counselor can play an important role in recovery as an active member of the treatment team.

ASSESSMENT OF SEVERITY

Professionals would classify as alcoholic or chemically dependent a person whose chemical use results in significant impairment in one or more of the following areas: spiritual health, emotional health, physical well-being, financial soundness, legal status, marital adjustment, and occupational stability. Early in the course of chemical dependency, relatively few of these areas would be affected. As the disease progresses, many more aspects of the person's life suffer. Severity is directly correlated to the extent of the consequences previously enumerated. Prior to manifest addiction, the person may be in the stage of "harmful involvement with drugs or alcohol." This designation is preferable to "alcohol or substance abuse," because it characterizes the person's harmful consequences without dealing with the issue of intentionality.

Substance *abuse* implies willful, clear-minded, intentional chemical misuse, a pattern which, seen later in retrospect, is actually the early phase of nonvolitional loss of control. Chemical dependencies are best treated at an earlier stage before widespread damage is done. Unfortunately, human nature being what it is, people tend to put off entering treatment until overpowering circumstances motivate them. Alcoholics are no exception to this rule. This does not necessarily mean that the outlook for recovery is poor, however. The best policy is to bring the alcoholic, no matter how seemingly resistant or hopelessly advanced, to treatment and keep him or her in treatment until it begins to take. In any case, it is best not to delay, since the disease is naturally self-perpetuating and can eventually be fatal.

CRISIS INTERVENTION

Simply stated, the best treatment program for an alcoholic is whichever one works for him or her. More severe cases characterized by extensive social disruption, physical manifestations of addiction, and impaired judgment require a multidisciplinary treatment approach beginning with hospitalization and medical detoxification. The goal is to place the person in a secure environment to interrupt the supply of alcohol or addiction-maintaining drugs. Then, detoxification is begun to prevent the onset of serious withdrawal symptoms such as seizures, hallucinations, tremors, anxiety, insomnia, vomiting, or confusion. Detoxification is usually accomplished by a tapering dosage schedule of tranquilizing medication. In general, the person is drug free in three to seven days unless severe drug dependency is present, in which case detoxification may take longer. The first step in crisis intervention means capitalizing on an alcoholic crisis and acting on the patient's or family motivation to put the person in an alcoholism treatment unit or under the care of a physician who specializes in alcoholism. Placing the chemically dependent person in a hospital setting or a secure, safe, sober treatment environment will double the chances of eventual success.

Crisis Intervention

Alcoholism is truly a "thinking disease," and the alcoholic will generally do best with specialized psychotherapy provided in chemical dependency treatment programs. These programs rely heavily on group therapy, often with recovered, previously chemically dependent counselors or volunteers. They almost invariably stress active involvement in the next phase of treatment, Alcoholics Anonymous (AA).

Involvement in AA cannot be overstressed if successful recovery is to be maintained. Indeed, the ultimate goal in chemical dependency counseling is usually acceptance of AA and active participation in it. Since most hospital alcoholism programs will orient the patient to AA, this work is usually done for the pastor. However, if the person does not go to a hospital, direct involvement with AA should be initiated, usually by having the person place a call to the local office of AA. Usually representatives from AA will visit the caller, offer to bring some literature, and escort him or her to a few meetings. In larger cities, the meetings are extremely varied, serving almost any social group or particular need. To be truly effective as a counselor for alcoholics and chemical dependents, the pastor should become familiar with the *Twelve Steps and Twelve Traditions* of AA (1981) and the "Big Book" of AA (1976).

The alcoholic will double her or his chances of succeeding if the family becomes actively involved in the treatment program. Most hospital units provide a good deal of family therapy and will attempt to involve the family in Al-Anon and Alateen, the family adjuncts of AA.

Antabuse is a prescription medication that acts as a deterrent to drinking by making the person ill if he or she drinks alcohol in any form. Not overwhelmingly effective by itself, Antabuse can be beneficial when combined with the comprehensive program described here. In any case, Antabuse is not to be taken lightly. Reactions with alcohol can be severe and even dangerous. If reaction occurs, the patient should be taken to a local hospital emergency room for observation or possible treatment.

At this stage, often in a hospital or in an intensive outpatient program, the pastor's primary responsibility is vigorous support of the treatment plan. Absolute abstinence from alcohol and mood-altering drugs is the rule. Resistance to compliance with any of these treatment recommendations should be viewed as continued manifestation of illness and impaired judgment, and the person should be guided persistently toward an attitude of full *surrender,* cooperation, and compliance.

Early stages of treatment involve considerable emotional and spiritual chaos. Early sobriety brings with it emotional instability, depression, insomnia, and irritability. Anger, impatience, and noncooperation are typical. Usually during treatment a process of self-evaluation occurs, an honest confrontation with the reality of chemical dependence and its consequences. Often a good deal of shame, remorse, regret, embarrassment, and resistance accompany this stage. Typically, however, an emotional catharsis is followed by a sense of relief, a letting go of resistance, and a sense of making real progress toward recovery. The pastor should do his or her best to facilitate honesty, openness, and willingness on the part of the alcoholic. Stigma, embarrassment, and self-blame should be avoided. People who suffer from diseases or disabilities are not blameworthy. The lesson of God's forgiveness and love should be repeated many times, and this phase will often culminate in dramatic spiritual renewal with an intense reaffirmation of previously lost spiritual values and attitudes.

COUNSELING IN THE RECOVERY PHASE

Recovery from chemical dependency is a difficult process. Two years of uninterrupted sobriety may elapse before real emotional stability and social restabilization are achieved. In the early period of recovery, the urge to return to chemicals will often be intense. The person suffers from addiction, and virtually any stress or emotional turbulence will trigger a desire for chemical use. Thus, the chemically dependent person must learn new, nonchemically assisted ways of coping with everyday reality. Often the smallest tasks will seem insurmountable obstacles to the recovering person, so support, encouragement, and actual physical assistance will be appreciated. Of course, continued abstinence from alcohol and drugs should be encouraged. Associations with chemically involved former friends should be broken off. Very active participation in AA should be recommended. How often should the person go to AA meetings? A good rule of thumb is about as often as alcohol or drugs were used. If the alcoholic was a daily drinker, then in the initial phases of recovery one AA meeting per day may be required. That may seem like a lot to the uninitiated, but we are dealing with addiction, and one day of freedom from chemicals is quite an achievement for a recovering addict. The most severe alcoholics may need more than one meeting per day. Most alcoholics get by in the initial phases with three to five meetings per week. A regular schedule is advisable after the person shops around and finds AA meetings at which he or she feels comfortable. It is advisable for the alcoholic to have an AA sponsor, that is, a "Big Brother" or "Big Sister" who will escort the person to meetings, be available by telephone when needed, and orient the new person to the program. Whether or not a sponsor is present, make sure that the recovering alcoholic has your telephone number in case of a crisis. It is always better to receive a phone call from the person before the temptation becomes overwhelming, rather than after a slip. If the hospital program has follow-up sessions, encourage the alcoholic to attend regularly.

Spiritual counseling for the recovering alcoholic can have a tremendously positive influence on the outcome and quality of the newfound sober life. Purity, honesty, unselfishness, and love are fostered by the AA program, and the pastor can comfortably endorse these virtues and reinforce their practical application to everyday life. Purity is a virtue that requires new application in the AA program. It requires the elimination of immoral sexual attitudes and behaviors, and the AA dictum of "men with men, and women with women" goes a long way toward avoiding complications. The patient should avoid emotional or sexual relationships within the recovery program. Such inter-sex relationships generally undermine recovery for both parties and often lead to disappointment and relapse into chemical use. Purity should be extended beyond these sexual concepts to the working of a spiritually vital, focused, prioritized, uncomplicated sobriety program. Coerced cooperation should eventually be replaced by willing and grateful involvement, and immoral attitudes and behaviors should be avoided.

Honesty is the cornerstone of successful recovery. Alcoholics who cannot be honest with themselves and others are dramatically worsening their chances for success. Acquisition of honesty is a gradual process that involves a heightening of awareness through education and sensitization. Partly, it is a process of taking the blinders off and facing reality in a courageous way. The disease, of course, inhibits this, and recovery involves getting away from euphoric recall to realistic, honest, sober reflection.

Unselfishness and love are closely related virtues that the chemically dependent person should cultivate. Diseases of addiction are characterized by self-will run wild to the point that the needs of others are forgotten, ignored, or not even perceived. Recovery involves reawakened awareness of others' needs and renewed commitment to meet one's responsibilities toward others.

Humility is an important virtue to stress in recovery counseling. Indeed, the first step of AA stresses humility in an indirect way: "We admit we are powerless over alcohol—that our lives have become unmanageable." Alcoholics must recognize their own helplessness in the face of addiction, learn to relinquish their willful stubbornness, and cultivate listening and cooperation. Dramatic, quick recoveries often prove temporary. True emotional, physical, and spiritual recovery is not a rapid process. It requires persistent application, work, and careful adherence to the guidelines. Complacency and overconfidence are serious dangers to a proper therapeutic attitude. Once the person feels that he or she "has it figured out now," or "doesn't need the program anymore," relapse often follows.

Gratitude is emphasized in the AA program because it is the very antithesis of resentment, self-pity, anger, or disappointment. It is an "other-focused" emotion rather than a "self-focused" one. It necessitates a process of positive rather than negative thinking which forces the individual to recognize that his or her glass is half full rather than half empty. Gratitude recognizes the workings of God and humans in the daily success of the recovery program. It recognizes the contribution of family, friends, and significant others, and it facilitates a right relationship with God as the ultimate source from which healing, vitality, and serenity emanate.

Serenity, a state of mind that is neither inappropriately elevated nor depressed, is the ideal encouraged by AA. Chemical dependents often suffer from mood swings. Depression, self-pity, resentment, and negative thinking have for years conditioned the person to seek chemical escape, comfort, or euphoria. The resulting roller-coaster effects of highs and lows have led to emotional chaos and self-perpetuation of the addiction. Serenity, with its quiet satisfaction and contentment, is the antithesis of emotional extremes and should be the recovering person's ardently sought emotional goal. A return to healthy self-esteem, as opposed to self-loathing and self-hatred, is based on the contented management of a stable life. The chemical dependent has to learn the painful lessons that courage, self-confidence, and self-worth do not come from a bottle of alcohol or pills, but are the result of persistent strivings for self-improvement and spiritual enrichment.

Spiritual recovery involves the revitalization of one's relationships with God, humanity, and self. Spiritual enrichment necessitates spiritual-mindedness and spiritual conduct. Spiritual revitalization is often the slowest part of recovery. Physical and psychological recovery happen much more quickly. Delay in spiritual recovery may reflect the terrible degree of spiritual disorganization and disability characteristic of these illnesses. In any case, the patient should "bring the body and the mind will follow." Church attendance, activities, and active contact with the religious community should be initiated as quickly as possible, rather than delayed until the recovering person is "ready for it." A patient, persistent, welcoming attitude from the pastor and the congregation is needed. Daily prayer, meditation, and reading should be encouraged. The AA program also stresses these things, so they will not be new to the recovering person. Start with the simplest prayers, such as the morning prayer, "God Help Me," and the evening prayer, "Thank You, God," as a means of structuring a return to simple, honest, spiritual renewal. Prayers for strength, sobriety, and gratitude should be shared with the recovering person. We see innumerable circumstances in which pastoral counselors, through adherence to these principles, help suffering human beings back to sanity and health. The alcoholic is often a challenge to our pursuit of love, patience, forgiveness, tolerance, and wisdom. Yet the persistent application of these virtues as part of the multidisciplinary, holistic health care team will often play a significant role in bringing about the recovery of the entire person—body, mind, and spirit—from the ravages of chemical dependency. Further readings related to the spiritual history of AA are included in the Suggested Readings section.

Chapter 5

The Person Experiencing Loss of Contact with Reality

OVERVIEW

The person experiencing loss of contact with reality has one of the most severe psychiatric disturbances. In psychiatric language, loss of contact with reality is called psychosis, and the person who suffers from it is psychotic. Loss of contact with reality implies severe mental illness or impairment, and most psychotics in this mental state are severely handicapped.

Loss of contact with reality, also called "impairment of reality testing," may appear in one or several forms in the same person. The symptoms may be anywhere on a continuum from the benign memory loss and mild confusion of old age to agitated paranoia with homicidal intent. Impairment may be acute, short-lived, and prognostically favorable; or it may be chronic, progressive, and prognostically ominous. The course, duration, and outcome depend on many factors, most important of which is the cause of the illness. In general the acute degree of confusion, agitation, paranoia, depression, or reality impairment does not correlate with course or outcome. The symptom picture at any one time is not usually an indication of the severity, length, or prognosis of the illness. Some of the most wildly combative, agitated, paranoid, confused individuals, when taken to an appropriate medical facility, may clear within a few hours and be sent home from the emergency room with no residual impairment and no likelihood of relapse. This is especially true with drug-induced psychoses, such as those caused by hallucinogens, marijuana, cocaine, or amphetamines. On the other hand, relatively subtle personality changes may be the first signs of an insidious, progressive mental illness that could last years or even end fatally.

The nature of the illness or the cause of impaired reality testing is most critical. Psychiatry recognizes five major types of psychosis: toxic metabolic, depressive, schizophrenic, manic, and organic.

TOXIC-METABOLIC PSYCHOSES

These altered states of awareness and judgment are precipitated accidentally or intentionally by drugs, whether taken for recreational or medicinal reasons. Typically, the onset of the altered mental state is within a few minutes to a few hours after the last drug ingestion. The resulting reaction may include paranoia, ranging from mild suspiciousness to frank delusions. Often the level of arousal is impaired, sometimes with somnolence progressing to coma, or, in the opposite extreme, euphoria progressing to violent agitation. Often these reactions are seen in young people who are experimenting with drugs or in people with medical diseases who are receiving legitimately prescribed medications with mind-altering side effects.

Case Example

Reginald is a twenty-six-year-old male who is found by police walking on the street with no shirt or coat at 4:00 a.m. When approached, Reginald is confused and his speech is garbled. He has no explanation for his behavior and does not know where he is. He does not understand that the police are questioning him, and he begins to resist and becomes loud and argumentative. At that point, his brother arrives in a car, looking for Reginald. The brother is oriented and speaks coherently, and tells the officers that Reginald has been abusing "wet," a combination of marijuana and formaldehyde that, when burned creates the drug PCP (phencyclidine), a powerful hallucinogen. Reginald does not recognize his own brother, and, because Reginald has a history of becoming violent on "wet," a decision is made for the officers to take Reginald to the closest emergency room.

Recognition

Typically such individuals are acting bizarrely in dress, manner, mood, orientation, and behavior. Their thinking is quite distorted, resulting in paranoia, extreme agitation, and violent outbursts. Often presentations may include giddiness, staggering, falling, or somnolence. A history of recent use of a street drug, alcohol, or prescribed medication is suggestive of the cause of the psychosis, but if no such history is available, toxicology testing of blood and urine should be done at the hospital.

Assessment of Severity

Toxic drug reactions manifesting loss of contact with reality are by their very nature severe. The course of a drug-induced toxic psychosis is unpredictable at onset. One can never be sure if one is seeing the maximal drug effect or if there will be progression to violent delirium, coma, or even death. For this reason, all drug reactions involving loss of contact with reality should be considered medical-psychiatric emergencies.

Crisis Intervention

Because of the emergency nature and unpredictable course of such toxic drug reactions, the affected person should be taken to the nearest qualified hospital emergency room for immediate evaluation and treatment. Although the great majority of these reactions will clear spontaneously with time, it is always better to be safe and have the assistance of a comprehensive medical team available, in the event that the toxic psychosis worsens and becomes life threatening. Although it has become popular to "talk people down" from a drug-induced "bad trip," it is our conviction that such talking down is better done in a hospital emergency room than in a nonmedical setting where life-support help or psychiatric services may be precious minutes away.

Once the pastoral counselor has assured the transportation of the affected person to the hospital or other safe environment, he or she should convey to the medical staff whatever historical information is available. If possible, this should include

1. a description of the person's normal personality,
2. the last time the person was in his or her usual state,
3. a report of any drugs or alcohol that the person might have ingested,
4. a description of the behavior observed in the toxic psychosis, and
5. the name of a responsible family member.

Although most hospitals can provide expert evaluation and medical treatment for a person with toxic psychosis, most emergency rooms are ill equipped to deal with a confused, agitated, disoriented, hostile, loud person under the influence of a toxic substance. Emergency rooms and medical evaluations are frightening experiences, even for people with normal reality perception. Under the influence of mind-altering drugs, an emergency room visit becomes a profoundly frightening experience to which the person may respond with noncooperation, flight, or assault. Ideally, out-of-control, fearful individuals in such a state should be surrounded by gentle, kind, patient, supportive personnel with smiling faces and gently restraining hands. Unfortunately, most emergency rooms cannot afford to have four or five people occupied with an agitated patient for hours and hours while a drug-induced psychosis clears. Most resort to the most expeditious and economical way of dealing with the matter: putting the patient in restraints. This is done by tying his or her hands and feet to the hospital bed. Almost inevitably the patient will strongly object to this procedure, and seeing a person in restraints can be heartrending for family and friends. The pastoral advisor who might jump to the conclusion that such a procedure is barbaric or unwarranted must remember that placement of the patient in restraints and release of a patient from restraints are medical decisions based on protecting the health and safety of the patient, family, and medical attendants. In the emergency room these decisions must be made by the attending physician. They are not decisions for family, friends, or pastoral counselors. It is certainly not humane to free a delirious, confused patient so that he or she can pull out tubes, strike an attendant, run away from the emergency room, and die in an exhausted coma. Usually, the patient is too disoriented and agitated to appreciate or tolerate medical necessities, and the emergency room staff is usually too busy with the requirements of other patients to be constantly at the bedside, reassuring the toxic person.

The pastoral counselor can be of great assistance in the emergency room. Once the patient is medically stabilized and secure, the pastoral counselor can act as a familiar face in a foreign environment populated by strange "white coats." He or she can act as a friendly advocate and interpreter of what is going on and provide talking down in the form of constant interpretations of reality, assurance that the person is experiencing a temporary drug effect, and calming influence against the irrational fears of the delirious patient. Talking down and calm reassurance may require repetitive dialogue over a period of several hours. Such dialogue is very concrete and specific:

> You are at the emergency room of the hospital. You have had a serious drug reaction. The doctors are trying to make sure that nothing serious happens to you. The drug reaction should be over shortly. The things you are experiencing are from the drug reaction and are not really happening. Your mother and sister are here with us. We are going to stay with you until this reaction is over. I am your friend, Pastor _____.

It is not productive to pay much attention to the hallucinatory content of toxic deliria. The themes may be paranoid, sexual, violent, depressive, or persecutory. It can be extremely misleading to "interpret" these drug-induced states since the drugs themselves often have such a disorganizing capability. Drug-induced reactions usually clear within a few hours or days. Hospital admission may be required for those who fail to clear within a few hours, or when a suicidal overdose is feared. Some drugs, notably hallucinogens such as LSD (lysergic acid diethylamide) or PCP (phenylcyclidine), can cause extremely long-lasting toxic psychotic reactions, sometimes taking weeks or months to clear completely.

Counseling in the Recovery Phase

After recovery from the acute toxic effects, the patient is often entirely back to his or her normal personality and behavior. Recovery phase counseling then follows along the lines of medical recommendations. If a prescribed drug was the offending agent, perhaps lowering the dose, avoiding intentional overdose, or using a different drug would be advised by the physician. If the toxic psychosis was the result of drug abuse with mind-altering chemicals, aftercare counseling for chemical dependency or drug abuse is instituted as described in Chapter 4. The long-term prognosis for most drug-induced psychotic reactions is good, as long as the offending substance is avoided in the future.

DEPRESSIVE PSYCHOSES

Depressive psychoses were described in detail in Chapter 2.

ORGANIC PSYCHOSES

An organic psychosis is a loss of contact with reality arising from a serious medical condition that affects brain function. Often such impairments represent structural lesions or deterioration of brain tissue. The changes may or may not be reversible; therefore, the prognosis of an organic psychosis depends on the type of brain disease or injury involved. The most common type of organic psychosis is senile dementia. Other common causes are tumor, stroke, injury, accident, and a number of central nervous system diseases.

Organic psychoses are typically of slow, gradual onset and are often characterized by confusion, disorientation regarding time and place, memory loss, and deterioration of normal personality.

Case Example

Kevin

Kevin is an eighty-six-year-old retired plumber, a widower who has been living alone for ten years, since his wife died. His adult children bring him to see you, reporting that he was able to carry on independently until recently. Now they have noticed a gradual decline in his faculties to the point that he is no longer able to fend for himself. On their recent visits to his home, the children were dismayed to discover rotted food in the refrigerator, dirty dishes in the cupboards, and dirt and disrepair everywhere. They found evidence of a small fire that their father had started by neglecting a burner on the stove. The house was full of trash that he had collected and stored, thinking that such objects would be valuable or useful to him someday. The yard and outside appearance of the house was neglected, and the neighbors were complaining about the general deterioration of the place. The children had been called by the police on three recent occasions when their father ventured out in his car and was unable to find his way home even though he was only a few blocks away. Of additional concern is Kevin's neglect of personal hygiene. He seldom bathes and then only with considerable prodding from his children. His children have noted a profound loss in his memory, especially for recent events.

Such confusional states, even when mild, represent serious impairment and a threat to independent functioning. There should always be a thorough medical, neurological, or psychiatric evaluation. A number of tests may be employed to assess functioning of the nervous system. These might include an electroencephalogram (EEG or brain wave test), brain scan or MRI (magnetic resonance imaging), skull X rays, and spinal fluid examination. Results of these examinations may help to determine whether the organic process is reversible or irreversible.

The pastor's role in this phase is to encourage the family to locate competent medical care for such an evaluation. Sometimes it is difficult for a family to know when to take the affected relative to the doctor. In these cases, it is helpful to remember that an annual or biennial physical examination is a good idea for anyone over the age of forty and certainly over the age of sixty. Also, any noticeable decrement in ability to function normally and independently should be cause for a visit to the physician. It is never advisable for a family to assume that decreasing mental capacity is the inevitable consequence of old age; in fact, most elderly people never become senile. Often mental impairment in the elderly is attributable to medication, trauma, intercurrent disease, tumor, or depression. Since some of these are potentially reversible conditions, medical consultation should always be obtained promptly when any deterioration of function is evident.

The pastoral counselor can be of great help and comfort to the patient and his or her family at this stressful time. People with organic impairment may recognize their declining ability to function and be profoundly frightened by the implications. Or they may have little understanding of the tests or the need for medical treatment. Kind, supportive visitations to the hospital bedside may be critically helpful in giving reassurance, allaying fear, and providing spiritual support for the person. The family, too, may be extremely upset. Mental deterioration in a loved one is always an alarming and sorrowful prospect. It is at once a partial loss of someone held dear and a subconscious reminder of the vulnerability of us all to sickness and old age. Also, many families are appropriately concerned about questions that such serious illnesses raise:

> Can our loved one live independently or does some other arrangement need to be made? Can we provide a supportive living arrangement, or is a professional residential setting advisable? Can such a humane residential facility be found? If so, is it affordable? Will the service and medical care be adequate? If we

take in the affected person, will our own home life be harmed? Will a professional residential placement result in an angry reaction from the affected person, or in a guilty, depressed reaction in our family?

Crisis intervention for the pastoral counselor appropriately addresses all these issues, assisting the family and the affected person in finding their own unique solution. Often the services of a comprehensive team are needed because of the complex issues involved. Once a decision is reached, the minister can be invaluable in aiding the adjustment of the affected person and the family.

Since many organic psychoses are progressive and irreversible, the term *recovery phase counseling* may be a misnomer and the designation *aftercare counseling* may be more appropriate. Often the organically impaired individual is confronted with a massive, wrenching realignment of his or her life, as necessitated by his or her declining capacities for independent living. The patient may have to sell his or her home, along with other cherished possessions. The loss of familiar neighborhood surroundings, pets, and friends also must be endured. The affected person must become resigned to increasing reliance on others. Such growing dependence is often a distasteful proposition to people accustomed to independence and autonomy. The pastoral counselor in aftercare can provide a friendly ear for the expression of reasonable grieving over these losses, and can encourage the person to develop an attitude of patience, tolerance, acceptance, and serenity, while enjoying small daily pleasures and focusing on gratitude for blessings bestowed by God throughout life. The minister can reassure the family that such adjustments, though temporarily painful, are necessitated by the reality of decline and dependency. Guilt or, conversely, anger and resentment in the family are destructive but commonly seen emotions that the pastor should elicit, understand, and moderate.

MANIC-DEPRESSIVE PSYCHOSIS

Manic-depressive illness, also called bipolar disorder, is a mental condition characterized by periods of normal or healthy mental functioning interrupted by attacks of manic hyperactivity or profound depression. Psychiatry recognizes three types: the manic type, the depressed type, and the so-called circular type that fluctuates between the previous two.

Case Example

Jerry

Jerry is a forty-three-year-old mechanical engineer with a local corporation. His wife, in a state of great emotional upset, calls you stating that Jerry has had "some kind of a breakdown" and is "doing crazy things." For the past three nights he has not slept. He went to numerous electronic stores and purchased hundreds of dollars' worth of electronic tools, equipment, and materials, but until today he refused to say what these were for. For the past three days he has been tinkering with this electronic equipment. This morning his wife found a letter addressed to her from Jerry saying that he had received a coded message from the president of his company while listening to the car radio. The message advised him that the company had been infiltrated by members of a foreign government and commissioned him to go on a leave of absence from work to develop a new military weapon. It further advised him that all expenses he incurred would be reimbursed, and that this new weapon technology would surely produce hundreds of new patents for which Jerry would be amply compensated, possibly with a share of ownership in the company. His wife is deeply concerned about the letter because the company makes a household product that is not at all likely to be the object of international espionage, and Jerry barely knows the president of the company and has no experience with weapons technology. Additionally alarming are Jerry's further purchases. He decided to "lay in provisions" and ordered several hundred dollars' worth of groceries delivered to the home so that he could work without interruption on his "top-secret" project. He also purchased three identical cars in one day, explaining that this was to foil any bomb assassination attempt. Apparently a would-be assassin would never know which car he was driving. When his wife spoke to her parents about this and returned home accompanied by them, she found that Jerry had barricaded himself in the house and would let in only her. Claiming that her parents did not have a "top-secret clearance," he prohibited them from entering. On the telephone with you, she mentions that she has been married to Jerry for only five years but that he has been entirely well during that time. When she discussed Jerry's behavior with his mother, however, his mother became very concerned, saying that Jerry had had a serious breakdown nine years before, which required three months of psychiatric hospitalization with several shock treatments. At that time Jerry had been profoundly depressed and was found in his garage with the car motor running, trying to kill himself with carbon monoxide fumes. He had written a note saying he had done nothing for humanity, and because of his neglect, thousands of people had died from starvation and disease.

Assessment of Severity

Manic-depressive or bipolar illness presenting in its acute form is a critically severe mental illness that almost always requires protective hospitalization and definitive psychiatric stabilization, including drug therapy and possibly even electroconvulsive therapy (ECT). Manic-depressive attacks may be characterized by drastic personality alterations, markedly impaired judgment, bizarre delusions, grandiosity, hyperactivity, and reckless spending sprees, or, conversely, by profound depression and overwhelming self-destructiveness. While in remission, between attacks of mania or depression, the person may function normally or even at a superior level.

Crisis Intervention

The pastoral counselor should use whatever relationship he or she has with the affected person to convince him or her to see a doctor for evaluation. In general, agitated, hyperactive, manic patients are very unwilling and uncooperative in obtaining psychiatric evaluation. It is perhaps better to suggest going to an emergency room to have a medical checkup. If this is not possible and the manic attack continues unabated, it is best for the family to contact a psychiatrist immediately, perhaps with the prospect of starting the judicial procedure for involuntary psychiatric hospitalization. Such procedures usually are not complicated but do vary from state to state, and every local psychiatrist is likely to be familiar with the procedure. Hospitalization is almost always essential in these acute attacks. Delay may mean allowing the attack to worsen dramatically, exposing the patient and family to considerable risk and possibly retarding the patient's recovery. Often the pastoral counselor will see that the family is stunned and frightened by the illness and can scarcely believe what is happening. Denial, which may be profound, may take the form of rationalizing the patient's bizarre behavior or harmfully procrastinating about obtaining definitive help. The pastor, recognizing this natural human response, should assist the family in locating psychiatric help immediately and possibly in transporting the patient to the medical facility.

Once hospitalized, patients with bipolar illness tend to present serious management problems to the medical staff. They are often angry, suspicious, and hyperactive. Threats and actual violence are not unusual. It may be advisable to obtain a brief consultation with the treating psychiatrist to offer your help in providing a reassuring and stabilizing presence to the patient. If the psychiatrist agrees that it might be beneficial, visit the patient and explain that you are only concerned about his or her welfare and are eager for the patient to return to his or her normal self and normal life. In order to do this, however, the patient must cooperate with the medical staff, take medications, and accept whatever treatment is offered. Often such treatment initially involves powerful medications to slow the manic attack or to relieve profound depression. Medications used to control mania may include the antipsychotics, lithium carbonate, anticonvulsants, or all in combination. At times isolation or even restraints are needed because of extreme agitation, violence, or self-destructive potential. Suicide precautions are often in effect. Visitors may be limited or even absolutely prohibited until some semblance of control is regained. Electroconvulsive therapy may be needed to halt the acute phase of the illness.

The manic attack may subside in days, weeks, or months. Once recovery begins, the patient is less hyperactive, sleeps through the night, and is less paranoid. His or her behavior is more predictable, and the possibility of violent assault diminishes. Delusional, grandiose thinking may quietly persist without being constant and without directing the patient's behavior. The dominant mood becomes more appropriate. Giggly euphoria settles into occasional jocularity and good humor. Anger, irritability, and verbal attacks settle into mild, sarcastic needling. Seclusion or restraints are no longer needed. The person may quickly move to higher privilege levels, including visitations at home and eventual discharge from the hospital.

Counseling in the Recovery Phase

Later in recovery or in remission, most patients with manic attacks have difficulty recalling the severity of their psychotic condition and, once discharged from the hospital, are eager to resume a normal lifestyle as soon as possible (often to prove they are well and that nothing was wrong in the first place). This denial of the severity of the illness may lead to poor cooperation and compliance in keeping follow-up appointments and remaining on medications. Once the acute manic attack has passed, the therapeutic mainstay for the prevention of further attacks is often lithium. Lithium repeatedly has been demonstrated to be effective in reducing the frequency and severity of acute episodes, especially of the manic type. Its effectiveness in preventing recurrent depressive attacks is not so dramatic. In spite of its demonstrated effectiveness and the relatively low incidence of side effects, most manic patients do not like the "slowed-down" feeling (not apparent to others) the medication gives them, and they are often eager to discontinue taking it. In recent years, anticonvulsant medications have also found growing acceptance for the treatment of mania. For this reason, effective aftercare counseling often involves repeated admonitions to the patient to continue following doctor's orders. Close coordination with the psychiatrist is highly desirable. If the psychosis has not completely cleared, and the patient is not yet ready to return to work, repeated admonishments to allow for more recuperation time are needed from the pastoral counselor.

Often, aftercare counseling is done with the family present. Reestablishment of normal family harmony and stability is a major goal of the recovery process. Often the disease has had a devastating impact on family relationships, and there may be a good deal of uncertainty about the future. The family should be counseled to be patient, that the attack will clear in time, and that with reasonable adherence to the medical regimen, future attacks are preventable. Of course, the safety of family members and of the patient must be reasonably assured through the acute phase of the illness. In time, medical help and spiritual direction are likely to result in a return to the preexisting family condition.

SCHIZOPHRENIA

Recognition

Schizophrenia is a psychiatric disease manifesting itself in a wide range of symptoms and having an uncertain clinical course. Schizophrenia is a widespread disease that affects 1 percent to 2 percent of any population group around the world. Yet in spite of its widespread occurrence, little is actually known about its cause, mechanisms, and treatment. Schizophrenia remains one of the great medical mysteries largely because the workings of the brain and nervous system are only dimly understood.

Fortunately, the past fifty years have witnessed dramatic improvements in psychiatric care for schizophrenia with the positive result that most hospitalizations are now fairly brief and are generally followed by a return to reasonably healthy social functioning.

Numerous theories for the etiology of schizophrenia have been proposed, including genetic predisposition, faulty parenting, stress, biochemical abnormalities, and foreign substances. Although each theory offers some advantages, none can account for the wide variability of disease manifestations. Current psychiatric thinking views schizophrenia as having a biochemical or physiologic basis with contributions from the factors just enumerated. As understanding of brain physiology grows, so too will comprehension of this baffling disease.

Psychiatry recognizes several different subtypes of schizophrenia, most notably paranoid, undifferentiated, schizoaffective, and catatonic.

Case Examples

John—Paranoid Schizophrenia

John is a twenty-six-year-old unemployed male who comes to your home in an agitated state. The youngest son of a family in your parish, he has been in a psychiatric hospital for eight years. John is carrying a large briefcase with him, and he says that he wants to warn you about the "impending international crisis" that he smilingly states will result in "all-out nuclear war between the superpowers." He claims that he has become aware of "top-secret communications from the government through highly sensitive radio receivers" that were placed in his teeth by agents of the United Nations Espionage Force. These radio receivers are undetectable to others, but it is clear that he has been "marked" because his eyes can no longer move as they once did. He says they are absolutely frozen in their sockets despite his efforts to move them. (You observe that his eyes appear normal and he seems to have no difficulty moving them.) He produces a variety of old, worn, handwritten letters, saying that the documents are self-explanatory and asking you to read them. Your brief reading reveals that they are a jumble of nonsense and grandiosity with recurrent themes of espionage, mind control by alien powers, subversion of the world's religions by unknown malicious forces, and repetitive assertions about secret radio transmitters in the teeth of unsuspecting citizens. There are numerous letters to various world dignitaries, including the president and vice president of the United States, insisting on a full investigation into his allegations. John admits that he has been in and out of psychiatric hospitals for the past eight years but claims nothing is wrong with him. He says he was most recently released three months ago, but the psychiatrists were part of the international conspiracy to silence him, and they had him on mind-control drugs for this purpose. He is determined not to take the drugs since leaving the hospital. He is now warning you of the impending peril and is enlisting your aid in launching an international crusade against subversive elements.

Emily—Undifferentiated Schizophrenia

Emily is a thirty-nine-year-old woman who lives alone in an apartment provided by her family. Her mother, though of retirement age, attempts to look after her and provide for her. Emily has never been able to hold any but the most menial job for more than a few weeks. The most occupational stress she could manage was working occasionally in the family grocery store, washing and stocking vegetables. She could do this only under close supervision and would soon become weak and tired and unable to continue. Despite several hospitalizations for nervous breakdowns, she has been under good control in recent years with the help of psychiatric medications. Her appearance is pleasant, albeit nervous. She seeks pastoral counseling and guidance regarding a romantic attachment. She recently became involved in a Bible study group where she developed an infatuation for a sixty-five-year-old man. The man appears to have taken a kindly, helpful interest in her, but did not demonstrate any affection or evidence of romantic interest. She, on the other hand, began to interpret his every glance, mannerism, or utterance in a romantic way. She began calling him on the telephone with real and imagined problems, looking for advice and help. Soon she was sending him letters confiding in all kinds of personal matters and hinting at her desires for a more intense relationship with him. She admits that he is married but adds that she is somehow aware that his marriage is in name only and that she is the person whom he secretly desires. Yet since he is a married man, she is concerned about the morality of her desires and seeks your guidance. You phone her sister, who informs you that the family has been concerned about Emily for several weeks. They are well aware of her intense interest and fantasies about the man and say that recently it has been "getting out of control." They know the man well and say that initially he received her letters and telephone calls charitably and with a note of benevolent humor. Gradually, however, as the calls and letters became more frequent and urgent, he became annoyed and distressed with her intrusions. The man's wife has also become less tolerant about the steady barrage of communications. The family reports increased concern because in the past two weeks she has been buying gifts for him. Initially they were tokens of gratitude. Then they became articles of clothing and eventually an expensive watch. The man returned all the gifts to her or to her sister and repeatedly wrote her letters requesting she not contact him anymore. Emily disregarded all this and attributed it to the coercive influence of his wife. The sister states that the family has just about run out of patience and that hospitalization may possibly be necessary. She adds that this pattern of fantasized romantic attachment is characteristic of her sister's nervous breakdowns. The family is currently planning a meeting to persuade her to reenter the mental hospital.

Bill—Catatonic Schizophrenia

You are approached by the parents of Bill, a twenty-two-year-old male. The family is well known to you through church membership. His parents say Bill has had a nervous breakdown while in the military and has been sent home to a local hospital for further treatment. They visited Bill at the hospital and found it impossible to communicate with him. He sat motionless for hours at a time, staring blankly ahead, oblivious to the presence of others around him. They have not heard him utter a single word, except for an occasional grunt, since the illness began. The hospital staff reports that Bill has little interest in activities of daily living and, because of his inability to feed himself, has lost considerable weight. The onset of Bill's attack occurred four months earlier. Prior to that time Bill appeared to be an entirely normal young man, quiet but active in sports and the church choir. The military doctors have told the family that Bill had a nervous breakdown immediately after a fight in which he and another young man had traded insults and blows. Evidently the other soldier was taunting him for his unwillingness to join in an evening of carousing. At first Bill was angry at the young man, and then he was depressed about being mildly disciplined for fighting. He quickly sank into a mute stupor with virtually no muscle movement, speech, or spontaneous activity of any kind. He was given a psychiatric discharge from the military. The family has come to you hoping that, since Bill knows you, you can break through his wall of silence and get him to talk.

George—Schizoaffective Schizophrenia

George is a fifty-two-year-old man brought to see you by his wife. Both have been members of your church for many years. You have noticed that George has not looked at all well lately. His personal hygiene has deteriorated remarkably, and often his clothing is inappropriate. Sometimes he will wear a heavy overcoat to church on a very warm day, or on a cold day he appears without any warm outer garments. He looks anxious and distressed and smokes heavily at the interview. His wife reports that he has been unable to return to his construction job for the past year. George was a good worker until approximately six years ago; since then, his performance has been progressively impaired. His wife says that the men on the job feel that he is unable to concentrate on his work, and he has nearly been involved in some serious accidents as a result. He seems quite forgetful and oblivious to what is going on around him. He will frequently break into uncontrollable crying spells and have to go home. His work attendance has dropped off markedly, and he had to be hospitalized four times in the past six years. His wife says that when he has an attack he is profoundly depressed, with feelings of worthlessness, hopelessness, and suicidal despair. He has little to say and will spend virtually all his time in bed. She admits that he is completely neglectful of his grooming unless she badgers him into bathing and shaving. She says that all this represents a profound change from George's normal personality. Prior to the onset of his illness six years ago, George was a quiet man, a steady worker who kept to himself. He has been under psychiatric care for six years, and presently he is on several medications for depression and nervous anxiety. He is not working and is currently on medical disability compensation for psychiatric illness. When questioned, George confesses to feeling hopeless and sad and seeing no point in living. He cannot elaborate further on his thoughts and asks that he be allowed to return home. At that point he merely repeats that he is tired and cannot talk any further. George's wife doesn't know what to do with him and hopes that you can talk with George and possibly figure out why he became this way.

Crisis Intervention

Schizophrenia is a serious disease, usually involving episodes of hospitalization and outpatient psychiatric supervision. There may be acute attacks wherein manifestations of the disease are more evident and out of control, and these attacks generally represent a psychiatric crisis or emergency. Because of evident reality impairment, schizophrenics are unable to be fully responsible for themselves, so hospitalization may be required. Crisis intervention in such circumstances involves recognizing the manifestations of the illness or the loss of contact with reality and then referring or transporting the person to the appropriate psychiatric facility for definitive treatment. If hospitalization is recommended, gentle but persistent encouragement to follow the doctor's recommendations is advisable. In the hospital, most acute schizophrenics are quietly out of touch with reality, and visitors are generally permitted. During visitations, structured activities are advisable, such as going for a walk, playing a game, or working on a craft project. The pastoral counselor should be attentive to expressions of psychotic or unrealistic thinking and, if the treating psychiatrist agrees, may gently try to reinforce a realistic outlook. This reality reinforcement may be done by acknowledging the feelings of the patient as real but gently questioning whether his or her interpretations might not be mistaken. Such reality restructuring works best in conjunction with a team approach to reality reintegration, coupled with appropriate psychiatric medications. Insight, that is, realistic awareness and acceptance of the illness, may not be present in the disease, so the patient may be unwilling or unable to cooperate with medical treatment. Support from the clergy for cooperation with reasonable psychiatric treatment is welcome. Most acute attacks of schizophrenia resolve satisfactorily with medication, time, and a reality-reinforcing, nonstressful environment. Some more persistent attacks, however, may respond only to dramatic measures, such as electroconvulsive therapy (often needed in catatonic schizophrenia). At times the disease is characterized by acute attacks and subsequent remissions, and at other times by insidiously progressive deterioration. Treatment of the acute attack is always directed at lessening the symptoms and attempting to restore the person to maximal healthy functioning. Since the causes of schizophrenia are unknown at present, treatment does not actually cure the disease but controls its manifestations and lessens the severity of symptoms until a natural remission occurs. Once this happens, medications are maintained with the hope of preventing a relapse.

Presently, the mainstay of treatment for schizophrenia is antipsychotic drugs or major tranquilizers. These nonaddictive drugs are not calmatives or sedatives for typical anxiety or nervousness. Instead, they work to modify the chemical imbalances in the brain of the schizophrenic. These work best against the agitation and excessive arousal that characterize many schizophrenics. The medications also help to prevent delusions and hallucinations and allow the fastest possible return to normal social functioning. Fortunately, some of the newer atypical antipsychiotic drugs help with so-called negative symptoms—apathy, withdrawal, and functional immobilization. Both types of antipsychotic medications represent a truly modern medical miracle and have been the single most important factor in the dramatic reduction of the number of inpatients in psychiatric hospitals in the past fifty years. Prior to the use of these medications, little except for humane incarceration could be done for schizophrenics. In spite of the miracles that these medications have wrought, patients often do not like to take them, partly out of unwillingness to accept their illness and the need for treatment, but also because the medications have some undesirable side effects. Among these are sedation, dry mouth, constipation, muscle stiffness, and, occasionally, constant abnormal chewinglike movement of the face and tongue. In spite of being powerful tranquilizers, these medications do not have the same euphoria-producing or narcotizing effects as the often-abused minor tranquilizers and sedatives. The antipsychotic major tranquilizers are rarely, if ever, abused for recreational purposes. In spite of the problems associated with these drugs, they are, for the most part, extremely safe and quite effective when used properly. Often patients will require high doses of these medications in the acute phases of the illness but need only minimal amounts (or none at all) when well.

Counseling in the Recovery Phase

Once discharged from the psychiatric hospital, the recovering schizophrenic needs help to achieve the maximal stability, self-reliance, and "normal" functioning to the level that he or she can reach, given the limitations of the illness and the requirements for its treatment. Since many attacks seem to be precipitated by stress, after-care counseling is directed at modulating stress in the person's life, cutting back on work or family commitments, and, in general, diminishing responsibilities for a time until maximal reintegration is achieved. If there are areas of emotional stress, such as repeated conflict with family, friends, or employers, such conflicts are best avoided and may even require geographic separation until stability, control, and emotional distancing are achieved. Counseling should emphasize practical aspects of recovering from an illness that impairs contact with reality and interferes with normal thinking processes. It should emphasize long-term psychiatric supervision with medication, if prescribed. Attempts on the patient's part to "go it alone" should be discouraged unless the psychiatrist concurs. Counseling should also be directed at restoring appropriate reality processing and judgment. It is never a good idea to endorse bizarre or delusional thinking, and often an appropriate response in the face of a persistent or seemingly immutable delusion is an impassive, non-endorsing acknowledgment such as "oh," "hmmm," or "I'm not sure about that." If the patient is at all open to discussion about his or her thinking or behavior, a helpful reality-orienting approach is warranted, with clarification of mistaken notions and directive guidance for appropriate behavior. Examples are directive counseling with regard to sexually appropriate behavior, dress, choice of friends, and living arrangements.

Two notable caveats apply. The first involves endorsement of excessive, bizarre, or delusional religious preoccupations. Regrettably, such excessive and inappropriate religious preoccupation is often symptomatic of psychotic disorders, and the most florid examples of this symptom can be seen in large cities where sidewalk "preachers" badger passing crowds with their hallucination-inspired ravings, constant threats, and exhortations. Other more subtle forms abound, and the pastoral counselor is well advised to watch for such inappropriate religious fixations in a person with a previous psychiatric history. Often these religious inclinations, although well intentioned at first, soon become pathological. The person may even come to believe she or he is in special contact with supernatural (or occult) forces and that her or his thinking and behavior are totally controlled by outside agencies. In such cases, the pastor is advised to avoid religious references, scriptural readings, or other religious activities, focusing instead on here-and-now realities in the temporal realm.

The other caveat concerns psychosis-induced violence. Although most schizophrenics are passive, subdued, quiet, and withdrawn, some are agitated, fearful, hyperexcited, and dangerous. A significant number of psychiatrists are killed every year as a result of contact with such patients, and the pastoral counselor is advised to exercise caution in dealing with patients manifesting hyperactivity, paranoia, and menacing threats.

As seen in this section, the spiritual side of schizophrenia may involve several factors, such as loss of hope; abandonment of faith; excessive, bizarre, delusional, religious preoccupation; and incredible distortions of commonly accepted religious beliefs. The pastoral counselor, by virtue of his or her position as interpreter of religious scripture and tradition, is in a unique position to provide practical, reality-oriented spiritual counseling for the recovering schizophrenic by reinforcing hope and faith where they are lacking and by reestablishing trust in the agents of God's healing ministry (physician, clergy, family, or religious congregation). The pastoral counselor can open the door for realistic faith and hope in the person's lonely struggle against the disease. Also, by modulating religious excesses, the pastoral counselor can, perhaps, enhance a more normal, less deviant lifestyle, allowing for better social integration and less rejection by others. If the schizophrenic person cannot tolerate the stimulation of attending church with the congregation, perhaps an individualized form of worship could be of help at home or in the church study for bible reading, prayer, and counseling as appropriate.

Chapter 6

The Person with a Personality Disorder

OVERVIEW

Psychiatry recognizes that each of us has a distinct personality, yet the term *personality* is difficult to define. We might say that an individual's personality is his or her unique blend of repetitive reactions, emotions, moods, behaviors, appearances, dress, thinking, and social interactions. Clearly, personality describes a matrix of internal emotional factors, thinking styles, and behavioral patterns that are seen as the individual adapts to the world. We define personality in response to the question, "What sort of person is this?" The answer encompasses the entire range of attributes, characteristics, and behaviors that the person exhibits.

How does an individual personality evolve? In all likelihood, this complex matrix is the result of numerous factors, some of which are genetically endowed at birth, and some of which are accumulated through nurturing and experiences in society. In other words, nature and nurture, plus accumulated life experiences, serve to mold the unique personality that each of us has. Natural or genetic attributes determine the physical characteristics of the body itself and play a significant role in eventual personality formation. For example, physical characteristics might include tallness or shortness, strength or weakness. Other inborn characteristics, such as shyness, aggressiveness, or "temper," might influence temperament. The basic organism with its natural attributes is then acted upon by societal influences, the earliest of which are childhood nurturing experiences, usually in the family setting with parents and siblings, where the future personality is molded further by the rewarding and inhibiting behavior of parents and others. Parents may choose to reward or inhibit flirtatiousness, physical aggression, verbal aggression, shyness, outspokenness, cleanliness, sharing, anger, and the like. The developing personality is further influenced by role modeling or "copying" of the personality styles seen in the nurturing family, as well as styles seen outside the family. Because these influences are constant, contradictory, and imperfect, their influence on the personality is a composite of good and bad, healthy and unhealthy, adaptive and maladaptive.

When the individual personality leaves the nurturing family setting, it encounters still another molding influence, i.e., the demands of larger society and of stressful situations. The individual must meet his or her own basic needs for food, clothing, shelter, security, survival, play, space, love, approval, self-respect, serenity, and reproduction in a highly competitive world of scarcity. He or she must cope with and adapt to an imperfect human world of virtues and vices, and favorable and unfavorable situations. He or she may be forced to deal with the gamut of human emotions and experiences, including love, anger, greed, fear, poverty, deprivation, frustration, opportunity, competition, jealousy, change, illness, abandonment, or death. In other words, he or she must adapt to and cope with the human world of imperfect institutions and imperfect people in an environment that may be loving, neutral, or hostile. The individual is then forced to adapt his or her natural attributes and learned patterns of behavior to a style of coping that leads, more or less consistently, to gratification of his or her needs—physical, emotional, social, and spiritual. Gradually, the personality emerges as a result of these influences and becomes a more or less stable, repetitive pattern of reactions, emotions, behaviors, thinking, attitudes, interactions, and dress. This personality inevitably involves mixtures of positive characteristics such as idealism, unselfishness, and virtue, as well as selfishness, jealousy, greed, and vice. All of us have these conflicting elements within ourselves in ever-changing proportions.

In general, personality patterns tend to be stable, repetitive, and predictable, with some changes occurring gradually with time and age. The personality patterns that people acquire by adulthood typically remain identifiable and consistent until advanced age exerts its own biological influence. Once the dominant personality pattern emerges, the tendencies and traits that mark the individual are frequently seen and are reinforced by the environment. These traits, by virtue of their usefulness to the individual, are constantly practiced and skillfully honed to meet his or her needs throughout life. The development, emergence, and utilization of these personality characteristics are, by and large, an unconscious process. Often the individual has only a dim awareness of being similar to or different from other people. Often he or she is unaware of the impact of his or her personality on others.

Personality traits are not necessarily good or bad per se. They are shaped unconsciously by a complex interaction between a dynamic organism and a changing environment. The adaptiveness of a particular coping style or personality trait may well depend on the situation or the extent to which it is used. For example, traits of self-confidence, independence, fearlessness, and aggressiveness might be highly adaptive for a fighter pilot. These same traits might not be so adaptive in another setting, for example, in postmilitary civilian life in a highly interdependent, corporate desk job. Some potentially desirable personality traits might even be incompatible or unattainable. For example, a high achievement orientation may be incompatible with a need to be liked by many people. Nearly every personality trait has utility in some circumstance. But since we have an imperfect and limited repertoire of coping skills and traits to bring to an unlimited variety of circumstances and situations, sometimes these traits are ineffective or self-defeating. To the degree that our familiar, repetitive coping styles are exaggerated, overreactive, inappropriate, or functionally ineffective, personality problems arise.

Personality disorder is a more or less relative term implying recurrent, maladaptive, or exaggerated coping styles. Individuals with personality disorders are not mentally ill, but are perceived by themselves and others as different, with recurrent, predictable problems of coping in specific social situations, such as marriage and work. Psychiatry recognizes and defines several specific personality styles or patterns of coping. Exaggerations of these patterns that are seen on a repetitive basis are termed personality disorders. This is not to say that such traits are abnormal or pathological per se. Most people have many, if not all, of these traits to a degree, but the person with personality problems will repetitively emphasize certain ones in inappropriate, ineffective, and exaggerated ways. Each personality style works well for the individual in certain conditions and situations; yet each style has its weaknesses and resulting problems. In this chapter, we examine several well-recognized personality styles with their typical weaknesses and problems. We also explore recognition, severity assessment, crisis intervention, and recovery phase counseling for each of these personality disorders. In general, treatment strategies favor directive counseling and limit setting.

The first three sections of this chapter describe personality disorders characterized by impulsiveness, self-centeredness, poor self-control, excess negative emotion, and recurrent problems in adjusting to the needs of society because of the interference of exaggerated character traits. The treatment strategy for these *uninhibited* or exaggerated character disorders is generally one of providing external controls and building internal inhibitions against immediate expressions of emotion and behavior. The uninhibited personality may be enmeshed in a life of total chaos and instability yet remain emotionally impervious to its consequences and to the suffering of others. In general, the people *surrounding* the person with an uninhibited character disorder are most distressed. These people can include spouse, children, parents, and employer.

In contrast to these poorly controlled, exaggerated styles, people having *inhibited* character disorders, such as obsessive-compulsive and dependent-inadequate personalities, tend to be typified by overcontrol and nonassertion of reasonable emotion and behavior. The counselor can adopt a more eliciting, permissive approach with such inhibited people while trying to moderate old habits of avoidance, overcontrol, and nonassertiveness. With inhibited character disorders it is the patients themselves who are usually most distressed. Family members and employers may be totally unaware of the repressed emotion and internal turmoil these people experience. The external facade is always one of control and emotional stability. Rarely is there any violation of social convention or legalities. The last two sections of this chapter examine two representative inhibited character disorders and the treatment strategies for them.

IMMATURE PERSONALITY

Case Example

Tom and Marie, both thirty-six-year-old members of your church, are parents of two children, ages nine and seven. Tom is nicely groomed and well dressed in a tailored, coordinated outfit. He is casual, relaxed, outgoing, and friendly. His wife, Marie, on the other hand, seems preoccupied, serious, and businesslike. Her clothing is neat but inexpensive, and she occasionally glances at the talkative Tom with an obvious sense of irritation. After some initial pleasantries, Marie announces that they have come for marital counseling, and that their marriage is in serious trouble. She says she is sick and tired of Tom's recurrent involvements with other women and his inability to hold down a steady, well-paying job. Tom fidgets nervously as Marie continues. She says Tom has always been a handsome, fun-loving man who likes a good time. Everybody likes him, and most people find him to be bright, attractive, outgoing, and engaging. She and her husband have been married for eleven years, and Tom has worked in various restaurants as a maitre d'. He usually works at night, and his wife reports that he has been repeatedly involved with female employees and patrons. When these involvements begin, he starts staying out later and later and eventually does not come home at all. Often she begins to receive calls at home from women asking for Tom. Sometimes the callers hang up when she answers. Friends have repeatedly told her that Tom is "no good," and that he has been seen with other women on numerous occasions. She has confronted him and threatened him many times before about this, and he always promises that it will never happen again. He breaks off the outside relationship and things quiet down for a few months, and then this cycle repeats itself. The most recent crisis was precipitated when Marie found an article of an unknown woman's clothing in her car. In addition, she claims that Tom has not been a consistent provider for the family. She works as a secretary in a law firm and feels that she has been providing the family with most of its stable financial support. Tom's work record has been erratic. He works for six or eight months in a restaurant, and then either the restaurant folds, or Tom has a falling out with the management and quits. He then remains unemployed for several months while looking for work. Marie reports that they have no savings and do not own a home because of his erratic work history. She says that they were just beginning to save toward a down payment when Tom impulsively bought her a car as a "peace offering" after he had been accused of infidelities again. Further questions regarding Tom's background reveal that in his early years, he was the youngest child in a well-off, middle-class home. He was his mother's darling, and she protected and spoiled him in his early years. Tom's parents subsequently divorced when he was a teenager, and Tom attributes that divorce to his father's involvements with other women. Tom was an average student, but his teachers always felt that he could achieve more. Bright but lazy, he spent his high school years partying. After high school, he entered the military but was discharged as unsuitable for military life after he impulsively decided to return home to his mother and remained AWOL for two months. Tom dated many women before he met Marie, who was herself a patron in a restaurant where he worked. After a few dates, Marie was "madly in love" with Tom, and she became pregnant. They married quickly, and Marie was initially extremely happy because of her feeling that Tom was such a handsome man and that she was lucky to have such a "catch." Her optimism about the relationship faded quickly, however, as she began to suspect that Tom was still seeing his old girlfriends. She says she does not know how many women Tom has been involved with over the years, but she feels she cannot trust him at all. Interestingly, she feels that in a way he cannot help himself avoid these involvements, and she recognizes that at times he really tries to do something about it. He never seems able to sustain these efforts, however. She feels that he is "too good-hearted," and that he tries to help people who are lonely or in trouble, with the result that he ends up being emotionally and physically involved. She also bitterly adds that Tom's mother blames her for any problems in the relationship, saying, "There must be something wrong with you if Tom is not happy and is seeing other women." Tom sits quietly through Marie's comments and does not directly deny her assertions. He tries to calm her with words of endearment, and then proceeds to explain away his behavior with various excuses. He does not deny that he has been involved with other women or that he has been an unstable provider. He says that he is an outgoing person to whom people naturally gravitate, and that he has a gift of helping people who are in trouble. He goes on to cite a few examples of lending one person money, helping another get a job, and getting a third out of trouble. He recognizes that he frequently gets "emotionally involved" in these relationships, which always seem to involve women, but he blames the women for their misinterpretation of his friendly helpfulness. He denies any active part in initiating the relationships and claims, "I've done all I can to prevent these emotional involvements, but they somehow always seem to happen anyway." He does not share his mother's view that Marie has been an inadequate wife. On the contrary, he says that he feels guilty that she has done everything possible to make the relationship work, and that he has not been a better, more stable provider. He feels that he is a victim of uncontrollable circumstances in his job history and blames the economy, the restaurant business, malicious owners, and "just plain bad luck" for his inability to hold down steady work. On further inquiry, he admits that absenteeism was involved in several of his dismissals. With regard to the present marital crisis, he claims that his wife is "overreacting" to an innocent situation. He says that he merely gave a woman a ride home from work in his car, and that she must have dropped the article of clothing while riding. He denies any wrongdoing in the matter, claiming that he "can't avoid seeing women in his line of work." Marie retorts that she has heard these excuses for years and that if he does not change his behavior and attitude with regard to women and steady employment, she is going to file for divorce. She hopes that marital counseling will avert a breakup, for the sake of their children.

Assessment of Severity

Although this couple seemingly presents with an acute marital problem, your background information reveals that their relationship has been profoundly affected by a longstanding repetitive pattern of personality and behavior. Tom's personality is similar to that of a misbehaving child—one who is both charming and self-centered. On the positive side, Tom appears to have a "winning" personality. People consider him affable, outgoing, handsome, charming, fun loving, and well intentioned. On the other hand, upon closer examination, his behavior is also characterized by irresponsibility, inconsistency, impulsiveness, shortsightedness, immediate need gratification, intolerance of routine, and violations of social and moral ethical codes. Although his behavior appears self-indulgent in the short run, in the long run it is hurtful and destructive to Tom himself and to the people around him.

Tom's behavior is supported by a variety of typical defense mechanisms. *Denial* of unpleasant or unwanted reality is prominent here in several aspects: denial of the reality of a recurrent pattern, denial of the reality of eventual hurt to self and others, and denial of failure of his past efforts to improve. He *projects blame* onto others, including the involved women, restaurant owners, the economy, and bad luck.

Tom also employs *rationalization* in providing himself with excuses for his self-indulgence. He says the women need him, and that he is only trying to help people who have serious problems. He excuses his constant exposure to temptation by claiming it is unavoidable in his line of work. Tom's tendency to defend his actions is supported by his mother's attitude, which also involves denial and projection of blame onto Tom's wife. Tom's wife herself has inadvertently fostered Tom's immaturity with a long-suffering, tolerant attitude. His problems have clearly been apparent for many years, but she has never taken a firm stand or given him an ultimatum before now. If they do not involve themselves in intensive counseling, a familiar pattern will re-emerge, with Tom promising to do better, "being good" for a period of time, then gradually relapsing to the same patterns of behavior.

Crisis Intervention

Tom is too comfortable to change his behavior. He secretly believes, "She'll get over it" or "I'd better be good for a while," but he is not realistically facing the possibility of the collapse of his marriage and the pain that this might entail. The counselor must recognize that until both parties are uncomfortable with the present situation, nothing lasting will happen. For this reason, the counselor must help the couple openly and realistically examine the long-term negative consequences, and use these to provide the initial motivation for ending the problem behavior and accepting help.

The counselor should attempt to use the pain of a crisis situation as a motivating factor for persistent involvement in a *long-term* treatment plan toward the attainment of stable goals. No improvement can take place as long as the destructive behavior continues. Therefore, if improvement is the goal, the person *must cease* the destructive actions. If he or she is unable to cease, either the motivation for improvement is not there or the behaviors are driven by such a strong compulsion that hospitalization and more intensive psychiatric treatment may be needed. Individual family members should be encouraged to look at their participation in the development of the present problem. Concealment, avoidance, minimizing, excusing, blaming, and tolerating are to be discouraged. The disordered person must be encouraged to *listen* to people for guidance and judgment. The counselor should maintain an attitude of concerned, hopeful neutrality, being objective and realistic, focusing on long-term consequences without oversympathizing with the patient or family members. The counselor is advised to identify as his or her interest the long-term well-being of all concerned. By all means, he or she should avoid the temptation to rescue, to overidentify with, or to support the alibis and blaming of the immature person. On the other hand, the counselor must avoid the temptation to be too harshly critical or morally judgmental. The counselor must recognize that he or she is dealing with imperfect human beings who are struggling with powerful emotions and inadequate skills at managing their personal affairs. A kind, loving, concerned, but firm attitude, such as one might have toward a problem child, is appropriate. If the person and family have a willingness to work, the pastor should emphasize that they must persevere in a counseling program for six to twenty-four months, possibly in conjunction with psychiatric outpatient therapy or a self-help group. In Tom's case, involvement with Sex and Love Addicts Anonymous (SLAA) might prove extremely beneficial. Little can be done without long-term commitment to this plan, but if they are willing to work with the counselor, long-term stability can be achieved.

Counseling in the Recovery Phase

While acknowledging the reality of a present crisis, the pastor should note that such crises have happened before, and that a fairly clear pattern of repetitive problems is evident. It is often helpful to identify the problem behavior as destructive. Although such behavior may indeed be immature, irresponsible, or indicative of defects of character, most people regard such pronouncements as pejorative and harshly judgmental. Identifying the destructive conduct as a repetitive behavioral pattern implies that the person can exercise a degree of control over it. Vague personality labels such as "immaturity" are too nebulous and ill defined for most people to perceive and control.

If an explanation is needed for these behaviors, "old habits" or "delayed maturation" can usually be cited as causes which are amenable to change. These factors are doubly important because they are within the immature person. They do not contribute to his or her temptation to blame unchangeable, external factors that can, in the future, be called upon to rationalize further misconduct. For example, if the therapist emphasizes improper upbringing as a cause, the truly immature person, when confronted with further problem behavior, can always say, "But I was the victim of an unhealthy upbringing, so what can you expect?" The counselor should avoid such pitfalls by always insisting that the person is responsible for his or her own actions and their consequences in the here and now, regardless of past influences.

The counselor should also emphasize that the person has had only temporary success in dealing with these problems without help. In some way the person is his or her own worst enemy and continues to make the same mistakes. The person must recognize that this behavior is destructive, that his or her own efforts have not been successful in modifying it, and that outside help is probably necessary for a while until new ways of thinking and acting become habitual.

Therapy for character disorders usually involves emphasis on positive moral values and virtues, such as honesty, unselfishness, purity, love, humility, self-control, and spiritual-mindedness. One must learn to think before acting, to avoid impulsiveness and self-indulgence, and to evaluate the long-term consequences of one's behavior. When confronted with temptation, one must ask oneself,

> Is it something I will have to lie about or conceal from others? Is it selfish or unselfish? Is it loving or hurtful? Is it helpful or destructive to my spiritual development? Have I asked others about it first? Have I prayed about it first? Am I succumbing to an impulse? Will it help me toward long-term goals of stability, pride, self-respect, and satisfaction? Am I exercising adequate self-control? Am I protecting myself from temptation? Am I taking significant risks? Am I unconsciously sabotaging my life?

Real values such as security, family love, occupational and financial stability, spiritual enrichment, and avoidance of legal trouble must be emphasized repeatedly. These values can be sharply contrasted to short-term thrills, self-indulgences, or sins.

In order to achieve long-term avoidance of problem behaviors, some progress usually must be made toward emotional distancing from so-called enablers, who support denial, rationalizations, and projections of blame. The person exhibiting destructive behavior must realize too that such enabling, while perhaps done out of love and protectiveness, usually has the effect of reinforcing the old behavior patterns. Similarly, avoidance of dangerous situations is important, because of the risk of facilitating disinhibition and self-indulgence. Such situations are often characterized by isolation, loneliness, sexual provocation, or alcohol use.

Although this program sounds a bit like "mortification of the flesh," one must remember that the suffering person is, in fact, defective in his or her ability to exercise normal self-control and must therefore overcompensate a bit for this lifelong inadequacy and develop protective behavioral insulation against his or her own vulnerability to relapse. A return to normal balance without great danger of relapse may take years. With the passage of time and the recovery of behavioral and emotional stability, real spiritual growth becomes possible. There is a distinct difference between "not sinning" and living a healthy, vital, active, spiritual life. This level of positive health is more difficult if behavioral relapse occurs, and frequent relapses are to be avoided by enlisting help *before* they occur.

SEDUCTIVE PERSONALITY

Case Example

Jean, thirty-eight, and Bill, fifty-four, are members of your congregation who consult you about "a marital problem." Bill is a hardware-store owner who has come directly from work wearing work slacks and a short-sleeved shirt with an out-of-fashion, slightly garish tie. He is somewhat obese and moderately balding. Extremely angry and upset, he claims, "My wife is driving my crazy!" Jean presents a different picture. Her hair is bleached blonde, and she is stylishly and excessively made up. She is wearing long, dark, false eyelashes, heavy rouge and lipstick, and powerful perfume. Her clothing is tight fitting, revealing, and provocative. Her shoes are spiked heels of the string-strap, see-through variety. She appears petulant and bored with the proceedings and sits in your office grooming her already highly polished nails. Bill reports that he is upset over an incident which occurred a few months ago. Bill invited his brother and sister-in-law to spend a few days in their home while on vacation. They did so, and it seems that Jean and his brother hit it off immediately and spent a good deal of time together. In fact, his brother's wife began to complain, and she forced her husband to terminate their visit prematurely. A few months after the visit, Bill noticed that their telephone bills contained several charges for long-distance calls made to his brother's city. When Bill asked Jean about these charges, she replied that she had indeed spoken to his brother, but only about possibly arranging a family reunion a few months hence. A month or two later, Jean told Bill that she wished to go out of town for a long weekend to visit her cousin, whom she had not seen in many years. Bill began to be suspicious and called his brother's wife, who told him that his brother, too, had told her that he intended to be out of town on a business trip. Bill and his sister-in-law concluded that their spouses were planning a secret rendezvous, and Bill decided to confront Jean. She vehemently denied any intention to meet his brother and began to cry, saying that she was extremely hurt that he would even think such a thing. The next day Bill found a hotel reservation confirmation in another city for the dates in question. This reservation did not support Jean's story that she was going to visit her cousin, who lived elsewhere. Bill became extremely angry and distrustful at that time, and decided to bring his wife in for counseling. Background information reveals that Jean is one of two girls born to a blue-collar family. Jean's mother had always wanted her to be an actress or a model, and Jean herself had little tolerance for school. She was briefly involved in dramatics in high school, but when she was sixteen she ran off with a twenty-seven-year-old man who became her first husband. She says she was pregnant at the time, and after the marriage he immediately lost interest in her and refused to get a job and support her. The marriage was annulled within a year. Jean worked at various waitress jobs until she married her second husband, who was a career military man. He was seldom in town since he was frequently on military assignment, but when he was, he drank heavily and was violent. Jean describes him as "absolutely paranoid" with jealousy, and she says he was constantly accusing her of cheating on him when he was out of town. He punished her for these activities by beating her up frequently. She had a second child by this marriage, which ended in divorce after seven years. Jean met her third husband, Bill, while working as a cocktail waitress in a bar. He was a patron who ate lunch there and stopped in occasionally for an evening drink. Bill admits that he fell in love with her immediately and that he impulsively divorced his wife and left his three children to marry her. This is his second marriage, but his earlier divorce hurt him financially, and he says that they are in serious financial trouble from Jean's overspending, mostly on clothes. He claims she has over 200 pairs of shoes and that he has never seen her wear the same outfit twice. He says that their sexual involvement, which initially was extremely exciting, cooled off quickly, and now Jean has no interest in him sexually. She refuses to allow him into the bedroom, and she has not permitted sexual intimacy for at least three months. Bill is extremely upset about her domestic irresponsibility. He says she is neglectful of the children and fails to discipline them, yet she resents it when he does. He claims the house is messy and that she seldom cooks or cleans. In fact, he has taken over most of the household duties. Most of the time she complains that she is too tired or depressed to handle these responsibilities. He adds that Jean is extremely jealous of other women and does not get along with them at all. She has no female friends, but she gets along with men extremely well, at least initially. If Bill so much as looks at a woman on television or makes a comment about her attractiveness, Jean flies into a rage, throwing things and even assaulting him. He says she is extremely insecure about her appearance and her own self-worth, and that she is constantly running herself down and comparing herself negatively to other women. When asked for her point of view, Jean says that she is very unhappy in her marriage and regrets having married Bill. She finds him "boring and dull" and not sexually satisfying. She feels that he neglects her and spends too much time on his business. She complains that, in spite of all the time he spends there, he does not make enough money to supply her needs. She has deep resentments about the financial and time commitments required by Bill's first family. She claims to be extremely embarrassed and depressed about being "dragged in front of the minister" today. She denies any improper behavior and states that he is excessively jealous for no good reason. She says that she has trouble sustaining interest in sex and admits that sexual intimacy has been a problem for her recently. She says she does not like it and claims "all men are animals . . . all they think about is sex, sex, sex." She feels that men are constantly making advances toward her without her encouragement. These advances only reinforce her low opinion of men in general. She feels that if there is a problem, it is entirely Bill's, and that he must spend more time with her and less with his business and first family. Bill vehemently denies that this is the problem or that this will change the situation. He says he has gone to great lengths to accommodate her needs and has taken her on several expensive trips and cruises to spend more time with her. He says he lavishes gifts upon her and her children and feels he has deprived his first family and his business of much-needed money in order to satisfy her wants. Bill admits that he is jealous, but claims that she has given him reason to be. He has gone to the extreme of checking up on her with telephone calls and surprise visits during the day, and he has even considered bugging the telephone or hiring a detective to monitor her activities. Both say that they are very unhappy in the marriage and wish that they had never married. On the other hand, they both feel a "powerful physical attraction" that keeps them together. Bill says that this is their second attempt at counseling. About a year previously, they had seen another clergyperson, and Bill terminated the visits when he began to feel that his wife and the clergyman were becoming emotionally, and possibly physically, involved. Bill says he wants to save the marriage since he has given up so much to achieve it. He says he is very much in love with Jean, but he cannot stand her flirtatiousness, seductiveness, irresponsibility, and lies. He says that if these do not stop, and if their marital problems are not solved, they will either break up or kill each other.

Assessment of Severity

Seductive personality disorder is more easily recognized and more common among women than men. While seductive men tend to be more aggressive and predatory, overly seductive women tend to exhibit a mix of dependence, anger, and self-indulgence. Because most cases are women, we have chosen to describe a female case here.

In its adaptive or healthier forms, the seductive personality style can be functional and rewarding. Women with healthier varieties of this personality are physically and emotionally attractive, open, and responsible. They may be aggressive, upwardly mobile, and pursue careers, or they may seek out aggressive, care-taking mates, such as professionals. In their healthier forms, they are extremely charming and use this power to charm for personal, family, and career advancement. Sexual adjustment is usually stable and healthy in these cases.

Mildly dysfunctional women are attractive but more openly flirtatious and gregarious. There is an element of impulsivity and unpredictability which is reflected in present seductiveness and a history of mild social instability. Often these women "do not live up to true potential" and have a history of conventional but unstable relationships. They are often less aggressive in attaining career goals, but might work as secretaries, waitresses in better restaurants, and other jobs that require modest schooling and preparation.

Moderately impaired women with this disorder are often from a more deprived background and have a long history of periodic life problems. They are more impulsive, irresponsible, and dependent. They frequently seek out irresponsible mates and may form relationships alternately characterized by self-centeredness and unreliability. They may have masochistic tendencies with long periods of tolerance of verbal and physical abuse, but the relationships tend to be long term. Job instability is the rule, but when they are coerced by financial duress, they can work in low-skill jobs for periods of time. Work adjustment may be problematic, with evidence of immaturity, tardiness, irresponsibility, sloppiness, and sexual provocation in the work area.

More severe cases are characterized by gross character instability. In such women it is often difficult to find any area of healthy functioning, and their life history is characterized by conflicts and maladjustment throughout. There may be a hostile or abandoning father figure and a hostile-dependent relationship with the mother. Such women are often extremely moody, irritable, dependent, and jealous of others. Often they have dropped out of school at an early age and can obtain only low-level jobs such as waitressing. Their poor work adjustment and instability often lead to frequent job changes. Many of these women are, on the surface at least, grossly sexually provocative and very promiscuous. They often select mates who have criminal or addictive problems of their own. Many have massive authority conflicts and cannot tolerate any limits being set on their behavior. The women often have a core of desperately low self-esteem, resulting in jealousy of other women, masochistic self-hatred, and impulsive, self-destructive acts such as drug overdoses. These acts can be genuinely self-destructive or they may be manipulative. There is often a history of recurrent, frequent psychiatric care, generally without lasting results. Typically, the woman stays in therapy only as long as she is able to control the therapist and avoid serious confrontation. When this is no longer possible, she flees, has a temper outburst, or displays her anger behaviorally by an overdose or relapse.

Crisis Intervention

Women with this disorder often do better in couple therapy than in individual counseling. The pastor should see the spouse frequently, if not at every session, and avoid being seduced by the charming patient. In some cases, sexually charged relationships are the only ones the woman can expect, understand, and develop. If there is a history of sexualization of professional helping relationships, this destructive pattern should be avoided, and such women should have only female counselors.

The counselor must recognize that often such a seductive person is a "child-woman" whose sexual provocativeness camouflages an immature, dependent, unstable personality. With such women it is often helpful to refer to a split personality: a "good" personality and a "bad" or immature personality within the same person. It may be helpful to emphasize characteristics of the "good" person by encouraging loyalty, stability, honesty, responsibility, unselfishness, and purity. The patient should be directed to function in that mode as long as possible. The crisis atmosphere may be softened by buying time and emphasizing repeated visits, perhaps six months of counseling and therapy in which termination is discouraged.

If there is realistic danger of violent acting out, or minimal self-control over behaviors that are damaging to self or relationships, then psychiatric involvement is advisable. Avoidance of violence is always the first priority, and stabilizing the relationship is the second. It is usually best to encourage the husband to meet more relationship needs, since sexual provocation is often a cover for child-like dependency. Such attempts might include frequent loving telephone calls, going out often, enjoyment of parties and friends, and gifts. In the short run, such gifts and tokens can alleviate considerable anger and may provide the pathologically insecure person with external proof of self-worth and reassurance that her needs will be met.

Counseling in the Recovery Phase

In long-term counseling for these women, it may be useful to continue to emphasize positive personality features and values, as well as future goals as a good wife and mother or a responsible employee. Such goals require setting limits on impulsivity, self-indulgence, and thrill seeking. The woman should be encouraged to accept responsibility for her sexual provocativeness. She should be helped to tone down her appearance to avoid allowing an overtly sexual appearance to interfere with family and job stability. It is often helpful to address her desperate insecurity and need to be liked. Emphasize wholesome achievement at home and at work as a means of achieving respect. Often a return to school or to a job builds self-respect and self-confidence. Encourage her to develop friendships with other women, finding areas of mutuality to talk about, such as children, husbands, jobs, or school. Cultivate an attitude of unselfishness and genuine love in the marital relationship.

Cultivate gratitude for the contributions of husband and children, rather than a self-centered attitude of unhappiness about perceived inadequacies or shortcomings. Emphasis on self-control is vital, especially when allowing negative personality features to emerge in response to an angry mood or a temptation. It is helpful to emphasize keeping the wild side of the personality under control, recognizing that it cannot and should not be totally extinguished.

Such women are often very irresponsible, and it is helpful to emphasize performance of small responsibilities, such as being on time, working consistently, paying bills promptly, spending time with children, cleaning, cooking, and shopping. These daily activities often seem painfully boring and unimportant to such women, and neglect of such duties is not perceived by them as contributing to their problems with relationships. Such irresponsibility is often rationalized by blaming the spouse and his inattentiveness. "If he'd pay more attention to me, I wouldn't mind doing all those things for him." The goal of counseling with a seductive woman is stabilization of marital and occupational relationships through setting limits on the provocative and irresponsible behaviors that characterize the more serious degrees of this personality disturbance.

PSYCHOPATHIC PERSONALITY
(ANTISOCIAL PERSONALITY)

Case Example

Frank is a forty-year-old real estate salesman who was sent to see you by his employer for "personality conflicts." The employer advised you this morning that he was going to fire Frank because he could not get along with others in the office. There were unexplained disappearances of money at work and fraudulent expense account statements, and petty cash requests, some of which were traced to Frank. Frank was described as a good salesman, but erratic with considerable absenteeism. He is well known in the real estate sales community in your town as an effective but unstable worker. He has worked in many jobs in different agencies in the city, usually for short periods of time. A consistent feature is that things go well for a while, and then Frank's temper gets him in trouble. He has frequently been involved in arguments with clients and employers, and previous employers have claimed that he has lost business and cost them money. This employer says that Frank has a "big ego" and is inconsiderate of others. He does not listen to anyone, is disrespectful, and makes derogatory remarks about others in the office. The employer has also been contacted by several collection agencies that are attempting to recover bad debts which Frank has accumulated. The employer feels that he can no longer trust Frank to manage company monies, nor to demonstrate a positive and professional attitude toward other office employees and customers. For these reasons he has decided to terminate Frank's employment. Frank admits that this is not the first time he has been in trouble at work. He recognizes that there is a pattern of arguing with supervisors and other employees, and he says that he "doesn't like to be told what to do." He also blames his boss who he claims is "an idiot who doesn't know anything about selling." He acknowledges that he has "a little money trouble," and that he is currently in debt for about $50,000. Some of this indebtedness was accumulated through impulsive credit card purchases, but some was the result of gambling debts from sports betting. Frank describes some of his former gambling associates as "real thugs who are telling me to pay up or else." Frank describes himself in his earlier years as a "wild kid" who was always in trouble. He was a poor student and a "discipline problem" at school. He fought with teachers often and was expelled from high school in the tenth grade. He describes his father as "a no-good bum, a deserter, a violent drunk." His mother is described as "extremely loving, the best possible mother; she would do anything for us." She recently divorced her third husband, and Frank feels a strong sense of responsibility for her welfare. After Frank was expelled from school, he entered the military, but was discharged as "unsuitable" after six months. Frank alleges that he had a nervous breakdown while in basic training and subsequently sued the Army for disability pay. This lawsuit was disallowed as the court was unable to document any bona fide mental disorder. After leaving the military, Frank had numerous sales jobs, the longest lasting eighteen months. He has frequently been unemployed and says that his wife is constantly nagging him about his inability to hold a job for any length of time. He has been married for twelve years and says that his in-laws have never liked him. At present, he is not living with his wife. He says she started going out with another man two years ago and eventually she ran away with him, taking their two children. He does not know their whereabouts but vows that if he finds her, he "will kill her and her boyfriend." She requested a divorce, but he is determined to fight it in order to make his wife as miserable as possible. When asked how he supported his family through his long periods of unemployment, he says that his wife's family helped out. Frank has a history of problems with alcohol and has been involved in several attempts at alcohol rehabilitation, including Alcoholics Anonymous. At present he feels he does not have a problem with alcohol and does not need AA. He admits to having had many legal problems in the past. He has had nine or ten charges of drunk driving, seven or eight charges of disorderly conduct, and one concealed weapons charge. He also says he was indicted for grand theft (embezzlement) seven years ago, but the case was dropped due to lack of evidence. Frank goes on to mention that he "fixed the case through the help of a well-placed relative and a few thousand dollars." Frank admits that his wife always objected to his friends, who were constantly in trouble. "My wife always called them a bunch of bums." According to Frank, he and his wife saw several psychiatrists for marital problems over the years, but they were "a bunch of jerks" who never helped him and "charged a lot of money for nothing." He says he took revenge by never paying their bills. Although Frank has been sent here by his employer, he feels he has no serious problems and needs no help. He blames the entire situation on his boss, whom he describes as vindictive and jealous of Frank's success. He sees no need for continued counseling.

Assessment of Severity

The majority of antisocial personality disorders occur in men. In healthier forms, psychopathic personality traits tend to find acceptable outlets in the sales world or in jobs that require persuasiveness with little accountability. In its milder degrees, a psychopathic personality may be reflected in a mildly unstable early adjustment in school with frequent, minor problems; however, these problems do not result in dropping out or being expelled. A person starting out as a problem child may manage later to find a niche and achieve a reasonably stable adaptation in business or private life. In moderately impaired cases, the individual may have a history of unstable adjustment at school, with truancy, authority conflicts, and rebelliousness. Later, work performance may be impaired by instability, impulsiveness, authority conflicts, and temper outbursts. Alcoholism may add to preexisting unreliability. In severe cases, there is marked maladjustment in all areas. There may be violent temper outbursts, often with minor provocation. Relationships with all authority figures and family members are seriously impaired. Police involvement and even a lengthy criminal record are common.

Crisis Intervention

General guidelines for the uninhibited personality disorders apply, but of particular importance is the need not to rescue or protect the individual from the consequences of his or her actions. Interceding to get a job back or mitigating legal punishment or prosecution are examples of possibly harmful rescuing. It is important to walk a fine line between being understanding and being sympathetic. Understanding implies the full realization of the behavior problems and attitudes that got the person in trouble, while realizing his or her need to correct them. Being sympathetic may put the counselor in the position of being manipulated against "persecutors" such as police, creditors, and lawyers.

It is important to be as calm as possible with these individuals, even though at times their behavior is extremely anger provoking. Acknowledge the person's point of view as sincere: "It may look that way to you, but others possibly see it this way." Referee and describe the conflict, but avoid taking sides. Emphasize the recurrent pattern of authority conflicts and violent temper. Absolutely prohibit violence of any kind and emphasize the need for self-control under all circumstances. Emphasize that there is no excuse for loss of temper or for displays of violence, antagonism, or intimidation. The counselor should certainly avoid exposing himself or herself to violence or risky heroics.

Hospitalization or jail may be necessary if there is immediate danger to self or others. If hospitalization occurs, generally group therapy in a supportive-confrontational milieu is best. Sedatives and tranquilizers should be avoided because of their high addictive potential. Such people do not like being "boxed in" and initially will not tolerate hospitalization. Pastoral involvement may help to keep the person in the hospital until the therapeutic process is established. Such people often do poorly in therapeutic relationships with authority figures such as medical doctors, psychiatrists, ministers, and others. Self-help groups are remarkably effective because of the absence of clearly defined authority figures, and because of their strong behavioral limit-setting approach. Groups such as Alcoholics Anonymous, Narcotics Anonymous, and Gamblers Anonymous are particularly recommended.

Counseling in the Recovery Phase

Such individuals are usually reluctant to participate in a long-term treatment contract. With external coercion from family, court, or employer, however, a long-term commitment may be obtainable. Long-term counseling repeatedly emphasizes accepting responsibility for one's behavior and its consequences. There should be emphasis on self-control, especially with regard to temper and impulsiveness. The person must try to accept imperfection in others and not be so easily angered by their behavior. He or she should try to acknowledge that the viewpoints and behavior of others are valid. An attitude of "live and let live" should be fostered. A counselor should emphasize personal stability and rigorous honesty in all things. This includes prompt payment of bills, discharge of financial responsibilities, and reliability toward spouse and employer. Lies (even minor ones), cons, or half truths should not be tolerated.

When a crisis appears imminent, the counselor should talk about the long-term consequences of psychopathic behavior or loss of control. Such consequences can include harsh legal penalties, such as lawsuits, fines, or imprisonment. Forthright discussions of the serious nature of these penalties will prevent the person from brushing them aside as tolerable inconveniences. Keep the person involved in counseling for six months or more and discuss all significant life decisions before any action is taken. Remember that this person has impaired judgment, and most tendencies, especially when stressed or angry, will be toward a relapse of psychopathic attitudes and behaviors.

Perhaps in no other character disorder is a spiritual program so therapeutically important. The person must give up grandiose self-will and self-indulgence and adopt an attitude of grateful humility, with an open ear for guidance from God and from other persons. Time should be structured as much as possible to avoid disorganization and the temptation to return to old habits or past times. Bible reading, counseling sessions, self-help groups, and organized church activities are recommended. Emphasize the daily performance of job and other routine responsibilities. Praise the person strongly for any accumulation of stable time, such as a month without missing a day of work. Put excessive energy to work helping others, such as working with juvenile delinquents or in Big Brother/Big Sister groups. Constantly focus attention on meeting the needs of others, such as spouse and family, rather than on self-indulgence. Emphasize virtues of honesty, purity, unselfishness, love, and humility.

OBSESSIVE-COMPULSIVE PERSONALITY

Case Example

Helen is a fifty-two-year-old housewife whose husband is a successful, busy upper-management executive in a local company. She arrives a half-hour before her scheduled appointment, which she arranged at your convenience so as not to interfere with your busy schedule. You recognize her immediately, since she has long been an active member of the congregation and has been heavily involved in boards, charities, and other church-related functions. She is (as always) meticulously dressed and groomed in conservative attire. In all your many years at the church, you have never seen her with a hair out of place, or with an outfit that was not conservatively color coordinated. Her clothing is comfortable, functional, moderately priced, and slightly dowdy, making her appear slightly older than her actual age. After offering some initial pleasantries and thanking you abundantly for your time and interest, she bursts into tears and describes herself as a "nervous wreck who can't cope anymore." She feels like a complete failure at home and is very guilty about letting everyone down. She says her husband and children are angry and upset with her, and that she has had difficulty controlling her moods and temper lately. Most recently, she had an angry outburst with her sixteen-year-old daughter, who refused to clean up her untidy room. This led to a shouting match, with Helen demanding respect and obedience and eventually slapping her daughter. Her daughter went to Helen's husband, and a family crisis ensued with everybody agreeing that she was becoming demanding, bossy, and fussy to the point that they could no longer tolerate her behavior. Although she feels some anger at her family members for their feelings toward her, she feels that they merely misunderstand her motives, and she insists that she is not trying to be bossy or domineering. She says that she is only trying to do the right thing and to raise her children with an appropriate sense of neatness, cleanliness, tidiness, order, self-discipline, and respect. She says this is more than a full-time job, and she feels a great deal of pressure as a result. She feels her husband, although he is a good provider, does not adequately supervise the children, and, in fact, is more of a "buddy" to them. She and her husband have had several long talks. Her husband complains that she devotes all her time and attention to household duties, such as cleaning and cooking. He feels that she exhausts herself to the point that she has headaches or mood changes, such as depression or irritability. She acknowledges that she works hard from morning until night trying to make a good home and a contribution to the community. She feels somewhat bitter that others do not pull their share of the weight, saying, "*Somebody* has to do it!" She wants you to intercede for her with the family to make them understand that she is only doing this for their benefit. Background information reveals that Helen is the oldest daughter of an upper-middle-class family in which the parents were extremely hardworking, religious people. They seldom argued, and Helen describes her mother's home as always immaculate. Helen's mother is still living and visits frequently. When her mother does visit, Helen feels extreme pressure and "knocks herself out" to make sure that there is not a speck of dust in the house or a thing out of place. Helen's husband has described her parents as serious, responsible, and hardworking, but rather cold and judgmental. Her husband once said, "They still have the first dollar they ever made." Helen was an excellent student who attended a religious college. She left after one and one-half years in order to be closer to her parents, and because she felt she was "not ready for school." She worked briefly as a teacher's aide and soon thereafter met her husband. She has three children whom she describes as "not very much like myself." She sees them as a bit spoiled but very outgoing, fun loving, and responsible. They have never given her much trouble until recently, when her sixteen-year-old daughter has become a bit more rebellious. Helen's husband is deeply involved in his work. She says that she is in charge of all the household responsibilities, primarily because "He doesn't do a good enough job on them." Her husband is not quite ambitious or hardworking enough to suit her. "I have to nag him a bit in order to get him to do things around the house." She feels she does not get adequate cooperation from the children or her husband in keeping her home orderly. Her husband feels that she has sheltered the children from learning responsibility by doing almost everything herself, seldom delegating chores or duties. The children always have their clothing laundered and pressed for them by their mother. Meals are always prepared and served without any help on their part. Helen says, "I can do it faster by myself." This visit was precipitated by her angry outburst with her daughter, as well as by recurrent episodes of tension-related headache and inability to sleep at night. She claims her sexual adjustment with her husband is not a problem, but she admits that she "can only get in the mood" after everything is in place and all the chores are done.

Assessment of Severity

In healthier forms, obsessive-compulsive traits are highly adaptive in society. Such people are punctual, frugal, hardworking, responsible, compliant toward authority, mannerly, quiet, and religious. They are often seen as highly responsible leaders in the community who will work hard for the church or other social causes. On the other hand, such persons have trouble with externalization of reasonable emotion and are not terribly spontaneous in having fun in unstructured social activities. They tend to be inhibited in expressions of affection and physical intimacy. In moderate degrees of dysfunction, such individuals suffer from exhaustion, depression, and self-righteous anger and disillusionment at the heavy burdens they feel others impose on them. Because of these internal and external stresses, they may have frequent psychosomatic or pressure-related illnesses such as headache, ulcers, spastic colon, and backache. They tend to be fretful worriers who have trouble sleeping. In more severe cases, overwhelming anxiety about the pressure of unmet responsibility may be paralyzing in its severity. Patients may experience depression, guilt, and feelings of worthlessness due to their inability to live up to self-imposed expectations. Other symptoms may include excessive, repetitive ruminating and worrying, checking and rechecking things to see that they are perfectly in order, and exhaustive attention to fastidious cleanliness and order, which, in more severe cases, may become pathological phobic concern about germs, bugs, disease, and contamination. Sometimes such individuals must pursue their activities in a rigid, ritualized, stereotyped fashion, following the same sequence of events without interruption. If an interruption occurs, they must start over at the beginning and repeat everything. Ambiguous situations without clearly defined guidelines for behavior are poorly tolerated. Situations that involve decision making and uncertainty are dreadfully anxiety provoking and stressful. In severe cases, such individuals make life difficult for everyone around them with their excessive preoccupation with order, cleanliness, and discipline, as well as with adherence to rules and social custom, strict dress codes, and religious observance.

Crisis Intervention

Obsessive-compulsive individuals often suffer from genuine depression, that is, from real feelings of low self-esteem, worthlessness, hopelessness, and unlovableness. In their most depressed moments, they are tempted to say, "Everyone would be better off without me." Your immediate task in a crisis situation with depressive overtones is to attempt to restore a sense of self-worth, recognizing the person's efforts to do a good job and make a contribution to home, family, and community. On the other hand, recognize that he or she appears to have taken this too far, past the point of usefulness, and perhaps to the point of unduly imposing his or her preferences on others.

It is often useful to acknowledge that these habits were programmed by earlier upbringing and parental values. Nonetheless, we must recognize the here-and-now reality that the patient is not living in his or her parents' home, nor should he or she be expected to adhere to the parents' supposed standards of cleanliness, order, and social appropriateness. Although cleanliness may be next to godliness, there is no moral or ethical imperative to be fastidiously neat.

Emphasize that the person's symptoms and distress are probably related to tension, fatigue, exhaustion, and depression from overdoing it and taking on too much responsibility. The pastoral counselor should say that the only relief from this suffering is through change, and then give the patient permission to accomplish this change. Granting permission is a very important counseling function with overcontrolled people. Such permission for even the slightest self-indulgence or brief whimsical irresponsibility often has not been granted to these people. They have been trained to a lifetime of self-discipline, self-sacrifice, and hard work, and the enjoyment of spontaneous, unproductive pleasure is seldom easy for them. Not only must the counselor give permission for enjoyment and for the putting aside of self-imposed burdens, he must also insist that these burdens not be picked up again and instead be delegated to others who are in a position to help, such as children, the spouse, a housekeeper, and others. Emphasize that the reward is better relations with children, spouse, and friends. It is impossible to be a pleasant, likable, cheerful person when one is exhausted, fatigued, worried, and resentful. To the greatest extent possible, the person must limit obsessive overdoing and worrying about small details in life.

Counseling in the Recovery Phase

In the recovery phase, counseling reinforces the principles just discussed. The person should be encouraged to relinquish the control and dominance that excessive compulsiveness creates and to avoid the angry feelings and consequent resentments that these behaviors engender. To the greatest extent possible, these people should be encouraged to relax, enjoy life, have more fun, take vacations, and avoid burdensome responsibility. Although this may sound hedonistic, in fact, these individuals will often have a difficult time tolerating even brief, unstructured relaxation time. The counselor must always try to prevent the recurrence of old habits of overdoing and overworrying on the part of the patient. He or she should enlist significant others in the person's life to accept the delegation of more responsibility so that they can help lighten the workload. Usually, however, the patient is his or her own greatest enemy in delegating responsibility. He or she feels that it is too much of a burden on the other people, that it would interfere with their lives, that they would not do a good enough job, and that the patient could do the job better and faster.

It is often useful to adopt a relaxed perspective toward such patients and their obsessive worrying. An attitude of humor and relaxed noninvolvement ("So what?") may free the person up from this self-imposed slavery of urgent responsibilities. After all, the world will not come to an end if there is a bit of dust in the house, or if the newspapers are not stacked and tied in a neat bundle. It is useful to encourage these people toward more spontaneous expressions of emotion, such as joy, mirth, gratitude, and affection. Getting them involved in singing or social activities within the church (without allowing them to dominate, control, or be victimized by their willingness to do the work) is useful. It is often advisable to curtail many of the outside commitments and community responsibilities that such people typically impose on themselves. If the person is extremely reclusive, however, getting her or him out of the house to engage in more social involvement may be productive.

Spiritual counseling should emphasize a loving, human, joyful, and spontaneous celebration of life. Prayer might be directed toward strength in the face of fear and anxiety. Humility should be stressed to counteract a strong sense of self-righteousness or self-importance. Such people are often judgmental about others and may in fact be "more religious than the church." The distancing effect of their attitudes upon others should be pointed out. Obsessive worriers should be helped to "turn things over to God," allowing Him and His infinite wisdom to work things out for the best. They need not feel that they have the burden of the universe on their shoulders, and they should allow room for the expression of God's will rather than their own in the affairs of humans.

Often it is important to free these people from the chains of perfectionism and the need to strive for the best possible performance or outcome. Often such striving is done only at the expense of emotional stability and positive relations with loved ones. It is far better to do an adequate job while maintaining an emotional energy reserve to meet other human needs. Often such people need permission to meet their own reasonable personal needs, for example, self-indulgences such as personal items, fashionable clothing, or other luxuries. There would seem to be little point in masochistic self-denial for no good reason and, in fact, such behaviors often merely earn the scorn of others. After all, nobody really wants to share life with a martyr.

DEPENDENT-INADEQUATE PERSONALITY

Case Example

Martha is a thirty-eight-year-old, unemployed housewife with five children. She comes to you complaining that she is overwhelmed with marital problems. She says her husband is a violent, irresponsible alcoholic who has been drinking recently and has frequently beaten her up. He has been seeing other women and not providing the family with basic support. Her bills are unpaid, and the utility companies are threatening to cut off services. She does not know her husband's whereabouts at the present time and has not seen him in three days. She has a six-month-old baby at home and is afraid of what might happen to herself and her children. She says her life has been hell. Her friends have all advised her to see an attorney and consider divorce, but because of her endless delays and indecisive helplessness, they are all fed up with her. Her husband's drunken, violent episodes have happened repeatedly in the past, and she has often threatened to leave him, but nothing ever comes of it. She always takes him back, and the same cycle repeats itself. Recently, her husband's violence has been directed more toward the children. In fact, juvenile authorities have come to the home and have threatened to take the children away if such abuse and neglect continue. Martha is a depressed, moderately obese, crying woman with a plain appearance, in a drab, soiled dress. Her nails are dirty, and she is neglectful of her grooming. When asked for background information, she says that her father was a severe alcoholic who was also violent and abusive. Parental fighting occurred, and she was a victim of child abuse and even sexual advances from her father. She remembers her father getting drunk and beating her mother. She did not apply herself in school, feeling that she was "too dumb" and that school was "too hard." She was an average child, well liked and dependable, and one who would "do anything for you." She does not consider herself a beauty. In fact, she recognizes that she is plain but fiercely loyal and dependable. She did not date much in her high school years but instead ran off at age fifteen with a sailor seven years older than herself. Her parents did not approve of him. They felt he was too wild and would not settle down. She thought that she could change him and that everything would be all right. She has had five children in this marriage, which has been interrupted by long periods of his unemployment and abandonment of the family. She says that she had children because her husband wanted them. Now that the children are there, he wants little to do with them. She feels that she is a helpless victim of circumstances and wants you to help her in some way. She requests that you talk with her husband to see if you can "straighten him out." Her life history reveals a longstanding pattern of inability to cope with responsibility or make realistic decisions in her own best interest. She appears to be excessively dependent on her husband and on institutions such as churches and hospitals to help her with her problems. She does not want to leave her husband "because I love him so much," and she asks, "What would happen to me and the children?" She continually makes excuses for his behavior ("It's just the pressure of not having a job") and habitually forgives and forgets his violence and irresponsibility. She is always forgiving, always tolerant. "He's really not that bad. It's not that bad for me or the kids."

Assessment of Severity

In mild degree, dependent-inadequate character traits involve little victim behavior. The person can participate in long-term stable relationships in which there is a dominant, protective partner. The resulting protection, security, and stability counterbalance the powerlessness and absence of control in these relationships.

Moderate severity involves more maladaptiveness. There is generalized failure to reach attainable goals, and more demonstrably poor judgment in mate selection and life choices. Long periods of "unstable stability," with depression, low-grade financial turmoil, and marital conflict, are common. Self-absorption and worrisome preoccupation with endless problems lead to neglect of children, with compensatory bursts of overprotectiveness.

In severe cases, there is a lifetime history of poor judgment and self-destructive behavior. Often the individual has a chaotic "life script" with a long history of maladaptiveness and misfortune. The person is often a poor student with a low level of scholastic attainment. She or he married early and badly to an abusive and/or neglectful spouse. Often, the mate or the patient abuses alcohol or other substances. Frequent violence occurs at home, with victimization of the patient or the children. The authorities may remove the children from the home. The mate is terribly irresponsible and may have severe psychiatric problems such as criminality, depression, or emotional instability. There may be a series of mates, all more or less alike in their innumerable problems. There are often many children and "overwhelming responsibilities" due to self-neglect and poor judgment.

The patient is often depressed and may have a long history of psychiatric counseling and hospitalizations. Often the patient has a history of frequent overdoses to escape reality by suicide, to manipulate a violent spouse, or to retaliate with self-destructive punishment for abuse. Such individuals may be heavily involved with supportive institutions such as hospitals, medical doctors, and psychiatrists. They are often unable to pay their bills and are always in a crisis of one sort or another.

Crisis Counseling

The home situations of dependent-inadequate people are often in great turmoil, with high potential for violence. The first priority is to protect the parties involved and avoid exposure to violence. The person should be encouraged to be strong and self-protective, as well as to set firm limits and stick to them. If there is danger in the home, the patient should call the police or at least go somewhere else until the danger passes. No one should be expected to live in a home with a threat of violence, abuse, or painful emotional neglect. Clearly, something should be done to alter the pattern of chaos and provide a stable, secure, loving environment for the children. It is often a good idea to separate the combatants until emotions subside. If there is no way to avoid violence, and the police response is not protective, hospitalization may be necessary for protection, stabilization, and to give the acute situation time to settle down. On the other hand, it is important to emphasize the lifetime pattern of chaos and victimization and to motivate the patient and spouse to seek help in changing the pattern. If either of the spouses is not interested in changing the pattern, and the relationship is not worth sustaining (it may be dangerous to the children), legal counsel should be sought.

Counseling in the Recovery Phase

Once the crisis has passed, the patient may be tempted to settle into complacency and once again succumb to the belief that "Everything will be all right now." However, nothing changes without extensive counseling and a good deal of effort directed toward change. The patient should be helped to develop awareness of the connection between the crisis events and to see that he or she is part of a pattern of passivity, helplessness, and excessive dependency on others. She or he should be admonished to cease "helpless" behaviors and stick to an ultimatum that the whole family must change. Often this process is best begun by fostering a degree of strength and financial emancipation. Insisting that the patient get a job is often therapeutic, since employment may help the person to be less dependent and gain self-confidence and self-respect. Long-term counseling and legal advice should be obtained. Patients should be encouraged to develop relationships with friends and family outside the home and to listen to

them and follow their advice. Patients need to face facts about themselves and about the destructive behavior in which both spouses participate. No excuses should be condoned for violence *or* passivity.
Patients must learn to be fiercely honest in talking about home problems. No lies, cover-ups, or self-deceptions that facilitate passivity
should be allowed. If the patient's self-deception is a problem, the
pastor should talk to family, friends, or social workers. They will usually see the truth of what is happening at home.

Often there is paralysis of will in dependent-inadequate people.
They have a difficult time making a decision and sticking with it without backing down. They should be encouraged to put the plan in action and stay with it for the long run. If the home situation is violently
out of control, leaving might be the best answer. Mobilization of
other institutional supports, such as police, child welfare, psychiatrists, other mental health professionals, and Alcoholics Anonymous,
is advisable.

A spiritual program can be very supportive to these troubled individuals. They can be helped to pray for the strength, courage, and perseverance to face their problems squarely and change their lives if
necessary. The person can pray for hope, not necessarily that things
will automatically quiet down, but that through work and perseverance a more stable and satisfying lifestyle can be achieved. Being a
good person does not necessarily mean being a victim or enduring
endless suffering. Positive mental health does involve an element of
"selfishness," i.e., the ability to act decisively on one's own behalf
and in one's own best interest when the need arises. Paralyzed passivity in the face of imminent danger is neither virtuous nor healthy. The
pastoral counselor should emphasize the needs of the children and
support the person's desire to provide a more stable home than she or
he experienced as a youth. The pastor should encourage the patient to
do whatever is necessary to provide this kind of stable, nonviolent
home situation for the children, even if it means requesting child welfare supervision within the home by an outside agency. The pastoral
counselor should provide support and prayer to overcome fear, isolation, complacency, and procrastination. He or she should avoid empty
sympathizing or endorsing inaction.

Of all the character disorders, this one is particularly difficult to
treat successfully. Often it seems that there is very little on which
to build. The person has seldom had any rewarding life experiences

and has little self-confidence or self-esteem. Options are severely limited after years of neglect and bad judgment. Job skills are few, and the ability to handle job-related responsibility is poor. Sometimes the best that a counselor can do is to prevent violence and further deterioration and see to the reasonable welfare of innocent children. In general, such persons need frequent contact with counselors and other supports, such as church activities, social service agencies, healthy friends, relatives, and others. A great effort is typically required to overcome years of passivity and self-neglect, and the temptation to do nothing is always present. Because of these factors and the violent potential within the home, frequent visits and extensive program involvements are the rule.

If there is a danger or history of violence or severe mental abuse, or if alcohol, drugs, or weapons are a factor in the present crisis, evaluation by a psychiatric specialist with possible hospitalization is in order. In any crisis situation, avoidance of immediate danger is the paramount concern. Most of all, one must remember that promises to do better have been made before, and that unsupported good intentions usually do not carry human beings very far. The old patterns and personality traits are powerfully ingrained and difficult to modify even with long-term counseling. The person and family must be held on a course of extended involvement in the counseling program.

Epilogue

In this book we have tried to share both psychiatric and spiritual perspectives in order to help the pastoral counselor in ministering to the mentally ill. The psychiatric component can and often does involve many of the doctor's tools: medication, hospitalization, regular treatments, and counseling. The pastoral counselor brings tools of another kind: faith, prayer, optimism, hope, forgiveness, virtuous living, scripture, sacraments, healing rituals, and comforting traditions. Other professionals on the mental health team bring their tools: social services interventions, psychological testing, and a variety of therapies to improve adaptive, healthy functioning. An effective treatment team allows the patient access to a variety of helping modalities, each tailored to meet his or her individual needs. It is our hope that the information provided in this book will enable the pastoral counselor to navigate successfully through the strange and sometimes daunting world of the mentally ill and to be a truly effective team participant in a holistic health care approach.

Throughout the book we have presented information and clinical vignettes based on our experiences with the most frequently occurring types of mental disorders. The perceptive reader can see from these vignettes that psychiatric disorders are extremely diverse in their presentation, and that treatment interventions must be *highly individualized* to the needs of the individual patient. One size does not fit all. Each person with a mental health problem has his or her own unique blend of thinking, attitudes, emotions, behaviors, stressors, genetics, cultural influences, and social circumstances that shape the expression of the disorder and promote and retard the recovery process. Each individual is, in effect, a course in psychology that the treatment team must approach with a fresh and open mind, not with preconceived or inflexible notions.

Helping persons who have mental disorders requires a blend of science, knowledge, skill, creativity, cultural awareness, and intuition. It is a high art that often takes years to hone and perfect. Few circumstances in the career of a pastoral counselor will present such formidable challenges. Yet the rewards are there; miracles of recovery can and do occur every day. The pastoral counselor can make an enormous difference in helping the mentally ill person move to a higher level, using spiritual tools and the healing contact of ministry to bring about a change for the better.

A word of caution: Beware the sudden turnaround, the breakthrough flash of insight, the newfound inspiration to turn one's life around. Recovery from a mental disorder is usually a long-term process, one that involves learning and practicing new emotions, thoughts, attitudes, and behaviors, as well as unlearning old, self-destructive habits and thoughts. Often there needs to be a drastic reordering of priorities, with altogether new ways of doing things. Good intentions can be formed instantly; lasting changes usually take time, effort, perseverance, and guidance. Keep that in mind when the turnaround is rapid and "miraculous." A slow, steady, *persevering* effort will win the race. Most people are hoping for an instant cure, but know within yourself that pastoral help with the mentally ill is best viewed as a long-term, gradual process.

Remember to be a team player in working with this population. Work *with* the psychiatrist, psychologist, social worker, counselors, hospitals, and agencies to surround the patient with as much help as possible. Rarely will the interventions of one person be enough to effect a recovery. We favor a "links in the chain" approach to the patient. The pastoral counselor should be one among many helpful influences, or "links," for the patient. To be more than that exposes the counselor and the patient to a possibly distracting, overly intense dependent relationship that will often end badly for both. It is best to retain a bit of humility and give credit to God and to the team of helpers in the drama of recovery. An additional caveat remains: Do not do anything to harm the patient. Doctors learn this admonition in their medical training: *Primum non nocere,* or "First, do no harm." The initially helpful and well-intentioned contacts the pastoral counselor may have with the patient can all too easily become distorted, harmful, and even criminal. A solid professional keeps a certain distance from the patient and does not let the relationship become too personal. The pastoral counselor is there to provide only pastoral counseling, not affection, money, shelter, or sex. Although it would seem obvious that these boundaries are not to be crossed, transgressions can all too easily occur in the context of rescuer/victim relationships.

Both parties can become so energized that emotional and physical intensity builds quickly. Be mindful of your boundaries, and ask for help and guidance from the other members of the treatment team if you feel your boundaries are crumbling.

Last, rejoice in your calling as a pastoral counselor in caring for those with mental disorders. The work in the vineyard is hard and slow, but the harvest can be bountiful. Suffering is relieved and lives are saved every day. Your impact can be enormous, as the needs are often very great. If possible, seek out opportunities to help the mentally ill as part of a health care team. You will find the work exhausting, frustrating, thought provoking, humbling, and enriching, in turns. You cannot help but be changed by the process, as we the healers are guests at the banquet of healing. As we labor in our vineyard, let us all reflect with gratitude on the opportunity to partake of this abundant feast.

References and Suggested Readings

References

Alchoholics Anonymous. *Alcoholics Anonymous,* Third Edition. New York: Alcoholics Anonymous World Services, Inc., 1976.

Alchoholics Anonymous. *Twelve Steps and Twelve Traditions.* New York: Alcoholics Anonymous World Services, Inc., 1981.

Erikson, E. H. *Childhood and Society,* Second Edition, Revised, Enlarged. New York: W.W. Norton and Co., Inc., 1963.

Freud, A. *The Writings of Anna Freud, Volume II. The Ego and the Mechanisms of Defense,* Revised Edition. New York: International Universities Press, Inc., 1966.

Freud, S. *The Interpretation of Dreams.* In *Standard Edition of the Complete Psychological Works of Sigmund Freud,* Volumes 4 and 5. London: Hogarth Press, 1953.

Low, A. A. *Mental Health Through Will-Training: A System of Self-Help in Psychotherapy As Practiced by Recovery, Inc.,* Twentieth Edition. North Quincy, MA: Christopher Publishing House, 1977.

Office of Applied Studies at the Substance Abuse and Mental Health Services Administration (SAMHSA). *1991 National Household Survey on Drug Abuse.* Rockville, MD: National Institute on Drug Abuse, December 1999.

U.S. Bureau of the Census. *Statistical Abstract of the United States, 2000.* Washington, DC: Government Printing Office, 2000.

Suggested Readings

Alcoholics Anonymous. *Living Sober.* New York: Alcoholics Anonymous World Services, Inc., 1975, 1998.

American Medical Association. *Essential Guide to Depression.* Pocket Books, 1998.

Beck, A. T. and Emery, G. *Anxiety Disorders and Phobias: A Cognitive Perspective.* New York: Basic Books, 1985.

Beck, A., Rush, A., Shaw, B., and Emery, A. *Cognitive Therapy of Depression.* New York: Guilford Press, 1979.

Berne, E. *Transactional Analysis Psychotherapy: A Systematic Individual and Social Psychiatry.* New York: Ballantine Books, 1975.

Black, D. W. and Larson, C. L. *Bad Boys, Bad Men: Confronting Antisocial Personality Disorder.* New York: Oxford University Press, 2000.

Burns, D. D. and Beck, A. T. *Feeling Good: The New Mood Therapy,* Revised and Updated Edition. New York: New American Library, 1999.

Ellis, A. and Haylor, R. *A Guide to Rational Living.* Hollywood, CA: Wilshire Books, 1973.

Erikson, E. H. *Childhood and Society.* New York: W.W. Norton and Co., Inc., 1963.

Glasser, W. *Reality Therapy.* New York: Harper & Row, 1965.

Gold, M. *The Good News About Depression: Cures and Treatments in the New Age of Psychiatry,* Revised Edition. New York: Bantam Books, 1995.

Gold, M. S. *The Good News About Panic, Anxiety and Phobias.* New York: Villard Books, 1989.

Goldberg, I. K. *Questions and Answers About Depression and Its Treatment.* Philadelphia: Charles Press, 1993.

Gorski, T. T. and Miller, M. *Staying Sober: A Guide for Relapse Prevention.* Independence, MO: Harold House, 1986.

Hazelden Foundation. *Hope and Recovery: A Twelve Step Guide for Healing from Compulsive Sexual Behavior.* Center City, MN: Hazelden, 1987.

Hazelden Foundation. *The Twelve Step Prayer Book.* Center City, MN: Hazelden, 1999.

Hemfelt, R., Minirth, F., and Meier, P. *Love Is a Choice: The Groundbreaking Book on Recovery for Codependent Relationships.* Nashville, TN: Thomas Nelson Publishers, 1989.

Kaplan, H. and Sadock, B. (Eds.). *Comprehensive Textbook of Psychiatry.* Baltimore, MD: Williams & Wilkins, 1995.

Klein, D. F. and Wender, P. H. *Understanding Depression—A Complete Guide to Its Diagnosis and Treatment.* New York: Oxford University Press, 1993.

Miller, Normal S. (Ed.). *The Principles and Practices of Addictions in Psychiatry.* W.B. Saunders Co., 1997.

Moskovitz, R. A. *Lost in the Mirror: An Inside Look at Borderline Personality Disorder,* Second Edition. Dallas, TX: Taylor Publishing Company, 2001.

Mueser, K. T. and Gingerich, S. *Coping with Schizophrenia: A Guide for Families.* Oakland, CA: New Harbinger Publications, Inc., 1994.

Perls, F. *Gestalt Therapy.* New York: Dell Publishing Co., 1951/1965.

Roy, C. *Obsessive Compulsive Disorder: A Guide for Family and Friends.* New Hyde Park, NY: Obsessive Compulsive Anonymous World Series, Inc., 1989.

Satir, V. *Conjoint Family Therapy,* Third Edition. Palo Alto, CA: Science and Behavior Books, 1983.

Torrey, E. F. *Surviving Schizophrenia: A Manual for Families, Consumers, and Providers.* New York: Quill, 2001.

Wilson, R. R. *Don't Panic,* Revised Edition. Harper Collins Publishers, 1996.

Index